"*Light: Medicine of the Future* . . . is a pioneering
relates points to a coming revolution in which
approaches will give way to far more effective gentle ones. The extraordinary
clinical facts he has assembled offer the best proof that, if implemented,
the revolution is no idle promise."
— Christopher Bird, coauthor of *The Secret Life of Plants*

"Jacob Liberman's pioneer thinking takes the wonder of light and light therapy
to a new level of insight by blending it with a deeper health wisdom and
spiritual understanding. I thank him for bringing this exciting new information to public awareness. It's a great book."
— Gabriel Cousens, M.D., author of *Spiritual Nutrition and the Rainbow Diet*

"Dr. Jacob Liberman's book on the human photocell is a long-overdue review
of the immense range of knowledge of the direct effects of light and color
frequencies on the human energy system. *Light: Medicine of the Future* will
stimulate interest among the healing professions, but, even more important-
ly, it will point us in the direction of why we came to be at the peak of evolution on this planet. It will certainly enhance our love affair with light."
— Christopher Hills, Ph.D., author of *Nuclear Evolution:*
Discovery of the Rainbow Body

"Drawing from ancient wisdom and scientific understanding of light, Dr. Jacob
Liberman integrates the biochemical, psychophysiological, and spiritual
properites of light. This book gloriously illuminates the remarkable healing
properties of light and ultimately teaches the reader how to use this ubiqui-
tous powerful energy in a profoundly curative manner."
— Dana Ullman, book reviewer for the *Utne Reader*

"Liberman combines what limited scientific data is now known about this
new, rapidly developing science of phototherapy with his many years of
personal experiences with his patients. The end results are amazing."
— John Ott, Sc.D. (Hon.), author of
Health and Light and Light, Radiation and You

"Light is one of the critical environmental factors in total health; indeed, 'the eyes are the windows of the soul.' This book helps provide one of those windows."
— Norman Shealy, M.D., founding president of the American Holistic Medical Association

"Dr. Liberman's book is a milestone forward concerning the therapeutic effect of light via the eyes."
— Fritz Hollwich, M.D., author of *The Influence of Ocular Light Perception on Metabolism in Man and in Animal*

"The planet has brought forth Dr. Jacob Liberman to give us new insight on the nature of wholistic healing and our new evolving health programs."
— Bernard Jensen, D.C., Ph.D., author and lecturer specializing in longevity

LIGHT
Medicine of the Future

LIGHT

MEDICINE
OF THE
FUTURE

*How We Can Use It
to Heal Ourselves NOW*

JACOB LIBERMAN, O.D., PH.D.

BEAR & COMPANY
PUBLISHING
SANTA FE, NEW MEXICO

LIBRARY OF CONGRESS CATALOGING-IN-PUBLICATION DATA

Liberman, Jacob. 1947-
  Light : medicine of the future : how we can use it to heal ourselves now
/ by Jacob Liberman.
        p.   cm.
    Includes index.
    ISBN 0-879181-01-0
1. Phototherapy. 2. Holistic medicine. 3. Light — Physiological effect. 4. Mind
and body. I. Title.
RM838.L53 1990
615.8'31 — dc20   90-748
                                                                      CIP

Copyright © 1991 by Jacob Liberman, O.D., Ph.D.

This edition of *Light: Medicine of the Future* is the first paperback edition of this
book. It was originally published in hardcover by Bear & Company in 1991,
ISBN 0-939680-80-7.

Bear & Company, Inc.
Santa Fe, NM 87504-2860

Cover illustration: Kathleen Katz & James Finnell
Interior design and selected illustrations: Kathleen Katz
Editing: Gail Vivino
Typography: Buffalo Publications
Printed in the United States of America by R.R. Donnelley

9 8 7 6 5 4

DEDICATION

I dedicate this book to my parents, Sonia and Joseph Liberman, whose lives, based on truth, integrity, support, and love, have served as the foundation for my own life. You have always been by my side. I thank you for my blue eyes, which have allowed me to look deeply into my life and its meaning, and for my name, Jacob Israel, which has given me a sense of purpose. To my children, Gina and Erik, who have been my most powerful teachers, I thank you for loving me unconditionally and supporting me through difficult times. Your hugs and smiles are God's nutrition.

PERMISSIONS

Thanks to Dorothy A. Bernoff for permission to quote from personal correspondence. Thanks also to Richardson & Steirman, Inc., New York, for permission to reprint adapted material from Dr. Richard Frenkel's forthcoming book, tentatively entitled *Overcoming Stress*. Thanks to Rainbow Canyon for permission to quote from personal correspondence. Special thanks to Celestial Arts, P.O. Box 7327, Berkeley, CA 94707, for permission to reprint an excerpt from *Notes from the Song of Life*, © 1977, 1987 by Tolbert McCarroll. Thanks also to Sam Biser of the Swannanoa Institute, for permission to reprint portions from *The Swannanoa Health Report*, issues 2 and 3, entitled "The Miraculous Health Benefits of Ultraviolet Light." Special thanks to Joy Franklin of High Mesa Press for permission to reprint an excerpt from *I Come As A Brother* by Bartholomew.

CONTENTS

ILLUSTRATIONS

COLOR PLATES

FOREWORD

I first met Dr. Jacob Liberman in 1975 while I was lecturing at an optometric conference in Miami that he was attending. Since that time, our relationship has developed into a regular and ongoing exchange of ideas, a sharing of our personal discoveries and mutual excitement about light and its effects on all living things. Jacob has been like one of the members of a relay team to whom I passed the baton and who is now running with it very fast, as well as passing it on to others.

In reading his book, *Light: Medicine of the Future*, I became completely fascinated with both his personal and professional stories. He comprehensively summarizes the scientific knowledge now known about this new, rapidly developing science of phototherapy and transforms it into understandable common sense. In addition, he points out some very important factors often overlooked by science, based on his own experience and case studies.

Modern researchers must realize that a review of the existing scientific literature on a subject is not a substitute for real experience. Too often, important findings are prejudged as crazy or considered merely anecdotal because they do not yet exist in the scientific literature of the day. Are we to totally discount our own abilities to see, hear, and feel our everyday experience, trusting only the findings of others who differ from us in their view of reality? Magellan, for example, discovered that the Earth was round only by *physically* sailing around it, despite the prevailing belief of the day that the Earth was flat and that a ship would fall off over its edge if it sailed too far.

Even today, discoveries are too often considered invalid unless they fit into the realm of "cold, hard science." Recently, the editor of a health-related newsletter sent a letter to a leading cancer-research center in New York City requesting copies of their research to supplement his understanding, with a check to cover their expenses. He also included a copy of his well-documented newsletter on the benefits of ultraviolet light, about which I had been consulted prior to its printing. To his surprise, he immediately received his check back with a letter stating that they refused to send him any of their publications because some of the work reported in his newsletter had been discounted by M.D.s throughout the world. It is difficult for me to believe that in 1990 scientists would refuse to share their knowledge with other interested parties based on a difference of opinion.

Life on Earth evolved under natural sunlight and has existed for quite some time under the full spectrum of light that it contains. Many prehistoric tribes and even entire civilizations worshiped the sun for its healing powers, using its full spectrum of light to treat physical and mental problems, a practice known as "heliotherapy." Yet modern scientific medical research now claims that sunlight is hazardous to people's health, and all sorts of special eyeglasses and sunscreen lotions are marketed to give complete protection. Major financial interests have come into play, sometimes making the truth even more obscure.

Unfortunately, the natural heliotherapy of the past has been replaced by many artificial approaches, such as chemotherapy. It seems as though many of today's therapies are in some ways like taking a magic pill. They will either eliminate the symptoms or numb the senses sufficiently so that the problem won't be noticed anymore.

As discussed in chapter 12 of the book, a car's engine requires fuel, oxygen, and a spark to create internal combustion, which makes the car run. The human body also requires fuel (in the form of food), oxygen, and a spark (in the form of light) to ignite the process of metabolism. If the ignition system of the car is not functioning properly, fuel additives will not solve the problem. The same is true in the human body. Vitamins will not solve the problems caused by a lack of the appropriate wavelengths of light necessary to create complete metabolism. There is no question in my mind that the visible portion of the spectrum as well as certain portions beyond, especially the ultraviolet, act as the ignition system for all human biological functions.

Combining his many years of personal and clinical experience with the frequently amazing results achieved by his patients, Dr. Liberman has developed a foundational model for a new medical paradigm. As

I observe the growth and constant evolution that has occurred in this emerging field of which I have been a part, I applaud the work of people like Jacob Liberman, who continue to carry the torch forward and believe, as I do, that light is the medicine of the future.

John Ott, Sc.D. (Hon.)
Sarasota, Florida
June 1990

Dr. John Ott is considered a pioneer in the field of photobiology. He is author of Health and Light; Light, Radiation and You; *and* My Ivory Cellar.

PREFACE

My close relationship with light began in 1974, when a powerful experience laid the foundation for my future direction. Seven-year-old Aileen was brought into my office by her parents for a vision examination. The young girl had been referred to me for evaluation and possible treatment of a lazy-eye condition. She had 20/20 uncorrected vision in her better eye, but only 20/200 best corrected vision in her poorer eye. Although I had been practicing optometry less than one year, my interest in vision improvement, beyond the mere prescription of glasses, led me to experiment with a new technique utilizing light to treat her particular condition. The technique consisted of flashing a light source into a person's better eye and allowing it to travel through the brain, eventually stimulating the opposite eye. Since the eyes are connected neurologically, I found that I could use the better eye to train its counterpart to see more clearly. Using this approach, I was able to improve the vision of Aileen's poorer eye to approximately 20/25 within 30 minutes. Although the initial improvement was not permanent, after five sessions Aileen's vision in the poorer eye reached 20/20 and remained that way. She is now 22 years old and still has 20/20 vision in both eyes.

That same year I had another stimulating experience. While at a party, I had my hands photographed by an innovative method known as Kirlian photography. This technique photographically reveals some of the energetic emissions from the body. The experience not only showed me that the body gives off light, but that by changing the way in which we use our minds we can actually increase, decrease, and/or direct the flow of the body's energy.

In 1975, I began to develop a vision improvement procedure that I called "open focus." I soon realized that this method affected a lot more than vision. The technique was based on a specific aspect of human behavior that I had observed for many years — behavior that deals with the way in which we habitually approach our life experiences and consequently learn. I noticed that most people were always *looking* for something specific in life and that in this process they missed everything they *weren't* looking for. Since it appears that most of life's revelations occur when we are *not looking* for them, I began to realize that the way in which most of us were seeing was only allowing us to view, and thereby experience, a *partial* reality.

Based on this awareness, I hypothesized that if we looked at nothing, perhaps we would see everything. Experimenting with this supposition in my own life produced dramatic results. In addition to expanding my field of vision, reducing my nearsightedness, improving my eyesight, reducing pain, and changing my point of view, it allowed me to see things that I never previously saw or even thought existed. My first discovery was that changing the way I saw occasionally allowed me to see auras around peoples' bodies. I then noticed that the air was not invisible, as I had thought previously, but in fact had visible energy that could be observed in both particle and wave form. These discoveries led me to realize that people are meant to see passively, not actively, and that our eyes are meant to see for us, if we let them. In other words, *vision is meant to be effortless.* We need to learn to view life in the same way we view a movie—without any effort. To put effort into an effortless function only gets in the way of its fluidity, efficiency, comfort, and performance. Unfortunately, most people habitually use much effort for seeing and therefore never see many of the visible miracles of nature and life.

As a result of these insights, I decided to stop wearing my glasses, and I began to actively experiment with the workings of my mind. The major aspect of my experiments dealt with the integration of my mind and my eyes. Specifically, I was interested in how people actually see and why they see that way. During the several years I spent investigating these questions, I came to a number of powerful insights. One of the most important was that if we allow our eyes to see for us as they are meant to see, they will always bring our attention to anything in the environment that is out of place or not flowing with that experience.

An example is the way in which an artist works. While producing a painting, he or she frequently steps back and openly gazes at the piece to get a feel for how it is progressing. Although the artist is not specifically looking for anything special, his or her eyes seem to direct themselves to anything that is obviously out of place. This not only supports my belief about how our eyes work, but seems to indicate that perhaps all of our sense systems, as well as our entire physical system, work the same way.

Soon I began to realize that there was great purpose in the way I saw and that anything I was intuitively drawn to was important and required my attention. I started using this experimental premise in my practice and discovered some surprising things. For example, while taking a case history I would gaze casually, with an "open focus," at the person with whom I was working. At first I noticed nothing, but after a few random gazes I began to realize that my eyes were being purposely led to certain parts of the patient's body. As I looked at these body parts, I noticed that something seemed to be stuck there and that the body's energy appeared to be rerouted through an adjacent area. Initially, I didn't understand the meaning of my observations, but as I questioned my patients I began to realize that their significant physical and emotional traumas seemed, not so coincidentally, to be located in those same body parts.

The wisdom of the body started becoming very clear to me. Soon, I began to trust precisely what I saw and would ask patients questions related to my observations. Their response was frequently one of amazement. They would ask, "How did you know?" Much of the time I didn't fully understand the information that I was receiving or even why I was receiving it. Nonetheless, a definite correlation seemed to exist between what I saw and what patients revealed. The foundation for a new knowing was being created.

Then, in 1977, a dear friend told me of his experiences with a specific form of light therapy called Syntonics. Developed in the 1920s, Syntonics therapeutically utilizes different portions of the visible light spectrum to treat, by way of the eyes, an array of bodily conditions. I attended one of the College of Syntonic Optometry's annual courses, purchased their equipment, and thus began my present life's work.

My first patient, my mother, had recently lost the vision in her left eye due to an optic nerve disease. The frightening aspect of this was that 25 years earlier she had lost part of the vision in her right eye from the same condition; and her mother was totally blinded by this same disease. Terrified by the dismal prospects, my mother submitted herself to six months of medical treatment by several top ophthalmologists in Miami, as well as at the Bascom Palmer Eye Institute. With no improvement, she was told to adjust to her new condition, as nothing more could be done for her. At this point, she could see only a few blurry fingers directly in front of her eyes and had totally lost her peripheral field of vision.

My research told me that the color turquoise acts as an anti-inflammatory agent. I had my mother look at a specific turquoise light in one of my instruments for 20 minutes per day. After four days, I began to measure an improvement in her eyesight. By the eleventh day, she was emotionally uplifted, feeling much better, and beginning to "see" things to her sides. On the twentieth day of treatment, she was able to read a four-inch letter at 20 feet — a massive improvement — and had regained 80% of the peripheral field of vision in her left eye. She also noticed a significant improvement in her right eye, which had been impaired for the past 25 years. From these miracles evolved my life and the work presented in this book.

What is important is not just that we use our knowledge and tools to be better "fixers"; rather, it is imperative that we "evolve" ourselves, integrating everything that allows us to become whole, more relational, and aware of our global community. Our task is to take in and utilize light so that we may merge with our true selves and our destiny, thus facilitating the healing of our planet. As each of us becomes whole, we radiate light — light from within — unimpeded by our self-imposed emotional and physical blocks. The medicine of the future *is* light. We are healing ourselves with that which is our essence.

ACKNOWLEDGMENTS

Many individuals have contributed in a wide variety of ways to the making of this book and the ideas it conveys. First, I thank Dr. Harry Riley Spitler, Dinshah P. Ghadiali, and Dr. John Ott for their courage in moving forward into the darkness of night and emerging with nature's rainbow.

I am deeply indebted to Dr. Larry Jebrock for telling me about the science of syntonics and convincing me to purchase the initial equipment necessary to get started on this new path. I am also very grateful to the College of Syntonic Optometry for opening my mind to the miracle of light and for teaching me how to perform magic with it.

Dr. Ray Gottlieb, Dr. Robert Michael Kaplan, Dr. John Downing, Dr. Charles Butts, Dr. Lowell Becraft, Dr. Christopher Hills, Dr. John Searfoss, Dr. Fritz Hollwich, Dr. Elliott Forrest, Dr. Amorita Treganza, Dr. Martin Birnbaum, Darius Dinshah, Dr. Bruce Rosenfeld, Dr. Russell Reiter, Dr. Gary Trexler, Dr. Alexander Styne, Dr. Dhavid Cooper, Dr. June Robertson, Dr. Richard Frenkel, and Dr. Larry Wallace have either planted the seeds in my mind, or watered and fertilized the soil they are planted in, so that multicolored flowers could sprout and smile.

I thank all the wonderful people who have come to me professionally and shared their lives with me, thus allowing me to learn from their wisdom.

I am especially grateful to those close personal friends and family who have held my hand as I have walked through the journey of my life and supported me in being all I can be. I love you Eva and Herb Finkel, Buzzy and Gayle Kaufman, Herb Ross, Frank Levinson, David ("Ili Ili") Kapralik, Paul and Myra Berger, Stephen Feig, Suzy Hailperin, Elio Penso, Jacqueline Valdespino, George Robinson, Truth Paradise, Brendan Roberts, Ron Lemire, Rose Kahn, Margaret MacCarron, Rainbow Canyon, Terry Levy, Vittor and Pat Weinman, Mona Naimark, Carmen DeBernardi, and Eli Muller.

Very special appreciation goes to Dorothy and Louis Bernoff for their loving support and technical expertise in the editorial phase of this book.

My publishers, Barbara and Gerry Clow, and their staff, I also thank for recognizing my vision, believing in me, and supporting me to go forth.

Finally, I offer a wonderfully uncontrollable smile and gentle hug for Sky Canyon, who convinced me that I could do it, showed me how, and held my hand through all the seasons of this book.

INTRODUCTION

Fasten your seat belt. You are about to embark upon a journey—one that may amaze you, teach you, stimulate your mind, and captivate you. You are going on a journey of healing with humanity's oldest friend in the universe: light.

This book presents the story of an ancient yet newly emerging science: the science of light. This science bridges the gap between scientific knowledge, intuitive knowing, health, and personal evolution, thus acting as a foundation for a new paradigm in healing. It ushers in a new era in medicine. Light, a nonintrusive, very powerful tool, resides at the core of the new medicine: "energy medicine." What will become very evident during the 1990s is that light is the basic component from which all life originates, develops, heals, and evolves. This has been expressed by wise sages and metaphysical texts of the past and present. However, we are about to see a new marriage—between the "intuitive" and the "rational" sciences—a marriage that is *bonded* by light.

There is no such thing as treating the body as a separate collection of "parts," to be fixed when broken. Human beings are the embodiment of light; our troubles and ills result from our inability to take in and use light as a launching pad from which to heal and evolve. In my private practice, I have seen literally thousands of times that this is true. Miracle after miracle has convinced me that this science of the future is an investigation of inner space rather than outer space.

Part 1 serves as a foundation. It describes the body as a living photocell, stimulated and regulated by light entering the eyes—"the windows of the soul." The eyes are the entry points through which light has its profound effect on the regulation of human physiological and emotional functioning and the development of our consciousness. This part examines the role of the pineal, the body's light meter, and how it assists us in becoming synchronized with nature and thus one with the universe. It explores the world of color and how we use color to heal, and introduces the concept of light as food—the nutrient that catalyzes biological combustion in humans, just as it catalyzes photosynthesis in plants.

Because of humanity's haphazard approach to life, we have set ourselves up to experience chronic *malillumination*, which, like the epidemic of *malnutrition*, creates major imbalances in our ability to function as healthy, whole humans. Modern technological advancements, such as most fluorescent lighting, sunglasses, tanning lotions, and our general indoor lifestyles, may in fact be harming us more than helping us.

Part 2 presents the works of some of the early pioneers who, ridiculed for their work and frequently thought to be mad, were actually such far-reaching visionaries that science is only now catching up with them. Over 50 years ago they suggested ideas and treatments that have only recently been investigated and applied clinically. Today, leading-edge, highly respected physicians and scientists are doing some of the most advanced research and performing many of the clinical applications in the therapeutic use of light. These present applications include the treatment of various cancers, clinical depression, stress, visual problems, premenstrual syndrome (PMS), sexual dysfunction, and jet lag. Part 2 also shows how light can effectively enhance learning abilities, reduce learning disabilities, strengthen the immune system, and even play a role in life extension.

You have probably heard or read recently about the harmful effects of sunlight and, specifically, ultraviolet (UV) light. This issue is explored in part 2, and a comprehensive view is presented. You will discover that, in fact, UV is one of the most biologically active and important portions of the electromagnetic spectrum. This part looks at many of the approaches science has taken in proving or disproving the value of our most powerful ally: light.

Light and color contain the essence of what humans attempt to gain by eating food and taking vitamins, and, in fact, act as catalysts for the absorption and use of these nutrients within our bodies. Although light is being researched and utilized therapeutically in a variety of medical and nonmedical fields, its most powerful role may lie in its ability to unlock and unclog the mind with great expediency.

Part 3 presents this new medicine as a holistic approach to healing the physiological, emotional, and spiritual bodies, thereby giving new meaning to the term *psychoneuroimmunology* (the mind/body healing connection). My work deals with healing the body and mind simultaneously as a direct effect of making the subconscious conscious, and thereby transforming old cellular memory into a new experience of enlightenment.

This part explains why we are open and receptive to certain aspects of our lives, why we are partially or totally closed down, or *allergic*, to other aspects of our lives, and the way that we act as each other's healing medicine — which I call "human homeopathy." Colors, specifically those with which we are most uncomfortable, can become our most powerful allies, and they can be used to access old unresolved emotional traumas, which, when brought to the conscious level, act as springboards from which we can pull out, by the roots, the weeds we call "disease." Light is the medicine of the future that will propel humankind into the age of enlightenment.

To support your own further investigation into this new medicine, I have also included listings of products, practitioners, treatment centers, and sources of more information.

LIGHT

MEDICINE
OF THE
FUTURE

PART ONE

*Let There
Be Light*

1

The Human Photocell

Have you ever wondered why we call the process of profound human evolution "enlightenment" or why the portion of the galaxy in which we live is called the "solar system"? Doesn't the term "solar system" imply that human beings are of, or derived from, the sun? Why do people frequently make statements such as "Lighten up" or "You light up my life"? How does *living in the light* differ from experiencing the *dark night of the soul*? Is it possible, as renowned physicist David Bohm states, that "all matter *is* frozen light"?[1] Could it be that our evolution, in some deep way, is related to our ability to take in and utilize light on a spiritual level as well as a physical level? These questions, and many others, are now being looked at scientifically, rather than just metaphysically or spiritually. The visions of clairvoyant sages of the past may not be so different from the scientific discoveries of the present. We are now in an era of accelerated scientific discovery, and the gap between scientific knowledge and "intuitive" knowing is gradually being bridged.

The idea of light as an integral part of all life and creation has been evident since the beginning of time. Sunlight, our major source and provider of light, warmth, and energy, not only sustains all *life* on Earth, but it sustains the *Earth itself*. It not only provides plants with the energy for photosynthesis, which in turn sustains the lives of all animals and humans, but also is the source of much of our knowledge, since most learning occurs by way of our eyes.

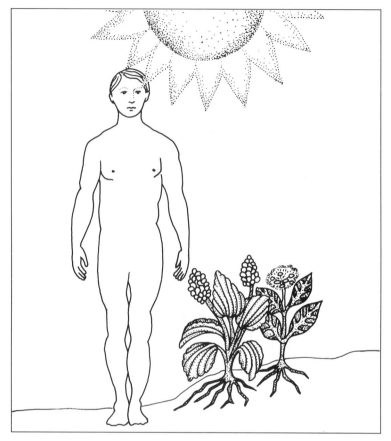

Figure 1. *Sunlight: sustainer of life.*

Sunlight is composed of a variety of energies that are transmitted to Earth in the form of electromagnetic waves. Only a small portion of these waves actually reach the Earth's surface, and only about 1% of the total electromagnetic spectrum is thought to be perceived by the eye. This visible portion of the electromagnetic spectrum, containing all the colors of the rainbow from violet (with the shortest wavelength) to red (with the longest wavelength) is a most important key to human functioning and evolution. Our lives, health, and well-being are truly dependent upon the sun.

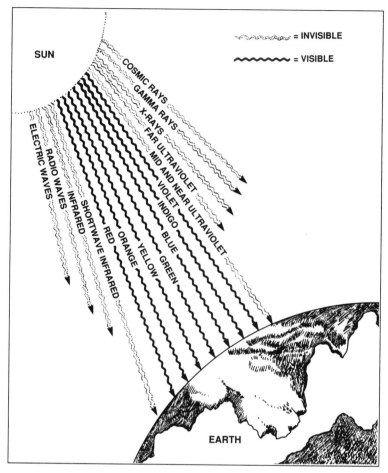

Figure 2. *The sun's electromagnetic waves.*

NIGHT AND DAY

When early humans first opened their eyes in the morning, they must have recognized that the light of each day brought with it a new beginning. Throughout history, we have recognized that this new beginning couples inspiration with increased physiological activity, heightened energy, and action. Each sunrise, a transition from the restful darkness of night to the energetic brightness of day, infuses life into all living things. (See color plates 1-4.)

Flowers open, animals and humans awaken, the world is energized, and a new day begins. Day is conceived and represented by the *yellow* of the sun, the *blue* of the sky, and the *green* of the Earth. As the day progresses, environmental color changes become evident, as well as their corresponding effects on all living things. The end of the day, beginning with the *red-orange* of sunset flowing into the *dark blue* of night, initiates a gradual slowing down of all physiological activity, followed by tranquility and rejuvenation. (See color plates 5-8.) The occurrence of this colorful transition from day to night dramatically represents the internal shifting of gears taking place within all living things. As nature gradually moves from one end of the color spectrum (red-orange of day) to the other end (dark blue of night), our bodies also shift from one mode of function (work) to another (rest).

Just as the shifting of gears in an automobile requires passing through the gear called "neutral," so this same phenomenon occurs in nature. Prior to the brightness of day shifting into the darkness of night, a well-known "flash of green" is frequently reported. Green, the center of the visible color spectrum, signifies the "neutral zone" or "drift course" through which all living things pass prior to entering a new phase of functioning or of life itself. From humanity's experience of the very first sunrise to the sunsets of the present, we continue to be awed by the beauty, power, life-creating, and life-sustaining properties emanating from light. It would appear, then, that our physiological and emotional centers are synchronized with nature by way of light, and that we truly seem to be the offspring of nature.

THE RHYTHM OF LIFE

Based on the awareness that daily color variations in the environment are intimately connected to the body's daily rhythmic changes, humans have recognized that seasonal color changes also reflect biological alterations within all living things. For instance, traditional Chinese acupuncturists, recognizing these biological alterations, routinely recommend treatments at the change of the seasons.

Thus, the seasons and their characteristic color changes have become a universal reflection of the role that color plays in different aspects of life experiences. (See color plates 9-12.) For instance, farmers have always known that there are different seasons for planting, growing, and harvesting. They have observed that seasonal variations and intensity in daylight control the budding, growth, and dormancy of plants. It is also apparent that animals are as involved as plants in this solar connection, inasmuch as their hibernation, migration, and breeding occur seasonally and thus appear very much related to changes in ambient lighting.

In humans, exposure to sunlight significantly influences a host of physiological and psychological functions. Among these, fertility and mood are two of the most profoundly affected. This can be seen in many northern European countries, such as Norway and Finland, where months of darkness occur annually. In these countries, a direct correlation has been found between decreased exposure to sunlight and a *higher incidence of irritability, fatigue, illness, insomnia, depression, alcoholism, and suicide.* Interestingly, it has been found that in Finland more children are conceived during the months of June and July, when the sun shines approximately 20 hours per day, than during the winter months.[2]

THE SUN: THE ORIGINAL HEALER

From the initial biblical statement "let there be light" to the idea of being "enlightened," light has played a consistent role in the development of all living things. The ancient Egyptians, Romans, Greeks, and other major cultures made significant medical uses of light. Although Egyptian physicians were the first to use color for healing,[3] the Greeks were actually the first to document both the theory and practice of solar therapy.[4] Heliopolis, the Greek city of the sun, was famous for its healing temples, in which sunlight was broken up into its spectral components (colors), and each component was used for a specific medical problem. Herodotus, the father of heliotherapy (a medical therapy involving exposure to sunlight) wrote that exposure to the sun is highly necessary in persons whose health needs restoring and who have need of putting on weight. In winter, spring, and autumn, the patient should permit the rays of the sun to strike full upon him; but in summer, because of the excessive heat, this method should not be employed in treating weak patients.[5]

Color, being a manifestation of light, held a therapeutic as well as divine meaning for these historical cultures.

MODERN SCIENCE RECOGNIZES THE VALUE OF LIGHT

The therapeutic uses of light have been known to many cultures for thousands of years. What are the effects of *light deprivation?* Probably the first direct reference in modern scientific literature regarding the influence of the sun's light on normal human growth is found in the book *Macrobiotics*, written in 1796 by Hufeland. He wrote, "Even the human being becomes pale, flabby, and apathetic as a result of being deprived of light, finally losing all his vital energy — as many a sad example of persons sequestered in a dark dungeon over a long period of time has demonstrated." Can you imagine how *you* would feel if every day was cloudy, with no direct sunshine? Or if you lived in a country with several months of darkness yearly? How about if you were confined to spending most of your time indoors? Isn't this, in fact, what most people do, and consider normal, from early childhood on? Could this possibly be the reason why people who work indoors frequently become overweight, pale, and lacking in vitality? Have we sentenced ourselves, through our lifestyles, to living as prisoners in modern-day fluorescent dungeons? As actor Tom Hanks says in the movie *Joe vs. the Volcano,* "These fluorescent lights are sucking the life out of me!"

More recently, Albert Szent-Gyorgyi, Nobel Prize winner and the discoverer of vitamin C, has recognized how profoundly light and color affect us. From his work he concluded that "all the energy which we take into our bodies is derived from the sun."[6,7] He saw that, through the process of photosynthesis, the sun's energy is stored in plants, which are in turn eaten by animals and humans. Digestion and assimilation by animals and humans are concerned with breaking down, transferring, storing, and utilizing this light-created energy.

Szent-Gyorgyi discovered that many enzymes and hormones involved in processing this energy are colored and very sensitive to light. As a matter of fact, when they are stimulated by selected colors of light, these enzymes and hormones frequently undergo molecular changes that alter their original colors. These light-induced changes significantly affect the power of these enzymes and hormones to cause dynamic reactions within the body. It also demonstrates that the apparent color of something might be a strong indicator of its molecular structure. Szent-Gyorgyi is saying that light striking the body can literally *alter the basic biological functions involved in processing the body's fuel,* which powers our lives. If color and light have such a powerful effect on us, what, then, might be the effect of living under light that is significantly different from sunlight? Perhaps this might be similar to the difference between running a car on inexpensive, regular fuel versus premium, high-octane fuel!

Similar conclusions were reached by Martinek and Berezin in 1979.[8] They found that light and color can play a remarkable role in how effectively certain enzyme systems regulate biological activity within the body. Specifically, they found that (a) some colors of light can stimulate certain bodily enzymes to be 500% *more effective*; and (b) some colors can increase the rate of enzymatic reactions, activate or deactivate certain enzymes, and affect the movement of substances across cell membranes. These findings seem to place light in a very powerful position as a regulator of many biological functions within the body.

Color may also indicate a person's stage of life or state of consciousness. I believe that light not only affects us, but that our state of consciousness determines how we use light. Consider how feeling ill seems to cause someone to lose all of his or her vital color, while embarrassment usually causes someone to become "red" in the face.

Perhaps the state of mind of these people has altered their ability to take in, utilize, and give off light.

The human body is nourished directly by the stimulation of sunlight or nourished indirectly by eating foods, drinking fluids, or breathing air that has been vitalized by the sun's light energy. This light energy not only affects our physiological activities and moods, but recently it has been shown to produce an effect in the body similar to that produced by physical training and its resultant improvement in physical fitness. Dr. Zane Kime, in his book *Sunlight*, states that a series of exposures to sunlight will produce *decreases* in resting heart rate, blood pressure, respiratory rate, blood sugar, and lactic acid in the blood following exercise; and *increases* in energy, strength, endurance, tolerance to stress, and ability of the blood to absorb and carry oxygen.[9]

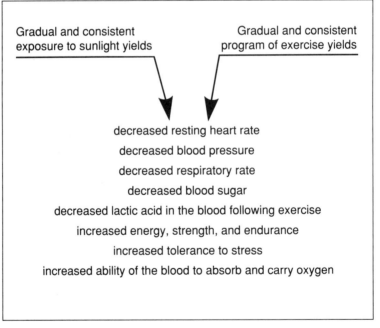

Figure 3. *Physiological effects of sunbathing versus physical exercise.*

In summary, these findings, along with those of many other highly respected scientists and physicians, seem to indicate that the human body is truly a living photocell that is energized by the sun's light, the nutrient of humankind. Since light is recognized as having a profound effect on all living things, and since our perception of light is by way of our eyes, it becomes evident that the function of the eyes may not be for "seeing" alone.

2

"The Eyes Are the Windows of the Soul"

— WILLIAM SHAKESPEARE

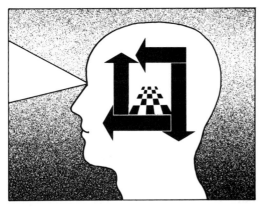

Figure 4. *"The eyes are the windows of the soul."*
Adapted from illustration by Elio Penso.

The eyes are wonderful tools for the examination and understanding of the universe, as well as primary sources of social contact and self-expression. Have you ever noticed, when you first meet people, how much their eyes reveal about them? If they're sad, their eyes will show it, and in the same way happiness and joy are immediately visible — by a gleam in their eyes. A person's eyes, as they subtly interact and synchronize with someone else's eyes, regulate the language of communication.[1] It isn't only the verbal interchange within a conversation that conveys a message, but the fluidity of the invisible dance

13

occurring between the two pairs of eyes that allows the communication to flow and conveys the feelings that are felt.

Shakespeare said, "The eyes are the windows of the soul." It is now
known that the eyes truly are a mirror of our physical and emotional
health. Acting as the body's Yellow Pages, they function as an accurate
index of what is occurring within the body and mind. Their examination can inform us of approximately 3,000 different functions or conditions pertaining to our physical health, as well as accurately indicate
our mental states and individual styles of operation.

WHAT THE EYES REVEAL

Light's relationship to the eyes as the major entry points into the
body and its subsequent effects on the development of our consciousness and consequent total functioning were noted quite early in history.
Most healers, including the great Hippocrates, have used the eye as a
window into the body to gain essential insights and assist their patients
in regaining health. The Bible states, "The light of the body is your
eye; when your eye is clear, your whole body is clear, your whole body
is also full of light; but when it is bad, your body is full of darkness"
(Luke 11:34). In 1856, Wimmer, an ophthalmologist at the Munich
school for the blind, clinically observed that "the youthful blind person
awakens as to new life if we succeed in enabling the eye to perceive
light again by removing a cataract or by forming a new pupil."[2]

Using the eyes as a microscopic map of the body, the nineteenth-
century Hungarian physician Ignatz von Peczely developed the foundation for the present-day clinical science of iridology.[3] He found that
the iris of the eye is literally a small map of the body. Present-day
iridologists utilize iris analysis to reveal abnormal tissue conditions,
inflammations, and toxic organs and tissues. They do not claim to
diagnose disease, but they utilize the appearance of the iris to evaluate
the body-tissue integrity, which, if not intact, is the precursor of any
disease. A December 1989 article in Soviet Life Magazine entitled
"Our Telltale Eyes" reported that Russian scientists, utilizing very sensitive video cameras, found a 100% correlation between the findings

of their newly developed iridodiagnostic technique and the actual physical conditions of the 150 subjects evaluated. Although many still consider iridology a pseudoscience, it has made great strides since the times of von Peczely and is continually being investigated as a possible diagnostic tool in the arena of preventive medicine.

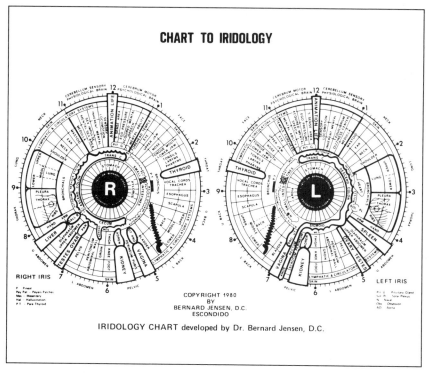

Figure 5. *Iridology chart. Reprinted with permission from Dr. Bernard Jensen.*

From this historical groundwork, it is apparent that strong relationships exist among light, our eyes, our health, and our moods. In order to understand the role that vision plays in our lives, a discussion of the eyes and their major functions follows.

THE EYES AND OUR WELL-BEING

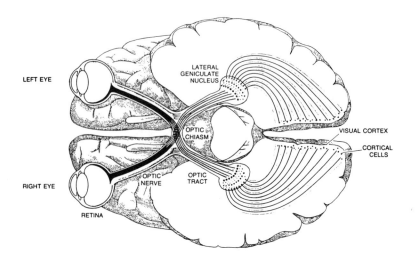

Figure 6. *The eyes are an extension of the brain. Illustration by Bunji Tagawa. Reprinted with permission of* Scientific American *from "Neurophysiology of Binocular Vision," by John D. Pettigrew, August 1972.*

The eyes, *which are actual extensions of the brain*, are more intricate and complex than any humanly conceived system to date. To illustrate this point the space shuttle Columbia, with its 5.2 million parts, could be compared to a single eye, containing 137 million photoreceptors and *more than 1 billion* total parts.

Although the eyes and brain represent only 2% of body weight, they require 25% of our nutritional intake. The eyes alone use one-third as much oxygen as the heart, need ten to twenty times as much vitamin C as the joint capsules involved in the movement of our extremities, and require more zinc (our intelligence chemical) than any other organ system in the body.[4] Housing 70% of the body's sense receptors, the eyes are the entry point for approximately 90% of all the information we learn in a lifetime (with the exception of blind people, who receive much of their knowledge from their other senses).

As a matter of fact, of the three billion messages relayed to the brain every second, two billion are sent from the eyes. The posterior third of the brain, which houses the memory bank and much of our intelligence, is also the portion of the brain used for vision.

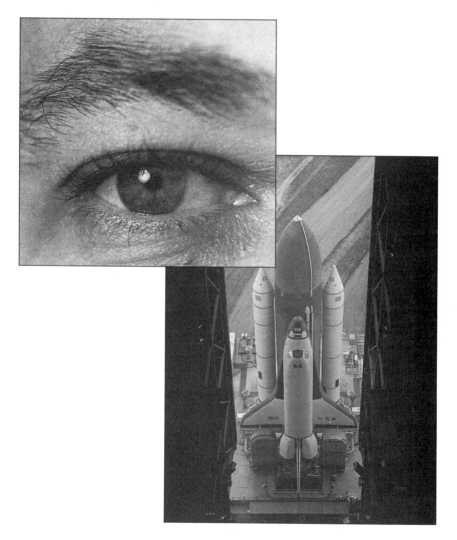

Figure 7. *The complexity of the human eye (more than 1 billion parts) as compared with the space shuttle Columbia (5.2 million parts). Photo of eye by Laura-Lea Cannon. Photo of space shuttle Columbia courtesy of NASA.*

Modern science is now beginning to look at the eyes as possible gateways to the mind. Some researchers are convinced that a definite link exists between eye color and behavior. They believe that different eye colors affect different areas of our brains, thereby influencing our personality and behavior.[5] If this is true, wouldn't it follow that merely looking at different colors would *also* affect different areas of the brain?

Another group of scientists have found that a significant relationship exists between visual problems and mental illness. Their findings indicate that while visual problems exist in only 9% of the general population, 66% of individuals suffering from depression, schizophrenia, or alcoholism have visual problems.

What, then, is really meant when someone is having problems seeing? Is the problem with the eye or the mind? In my own experience with treating thousands of people, I have found a significant correlation between the "vision" of the mind's eye and the corresponding vision patterns of the physical eye. During my sixteen years of practicing functional optometry, I have continually seen a significant relationship between specific mental patterns and the functioning (or dysfunctioning) of the eyes. I have noticed also that vision therapy is a very successful means of modifying patterns in both the eyes and the mind. This seems to substantiate the therapeutic value of using the eyes, and specifically visual patterns, as a way of diagnosing and treating the body and mind.

NEUROLINGUISTIC PROGRAMMING (NLP)

Recently, a new clinical science has emerged that looks at the relationship between eye movements and cognitive processing styles; specifically, it studies how people process and store information, and how their styles of processing manifest in their actions. This new science, Neurolinguistic Programming (NLP), was originally based on the clinical observation that eye movements seem to act as triggers to open up certain types of sensory recall.[6] If we conceive of the mind as being made up of many different reference libraries, each storing a certain type of experience, then what researchers have noticed is that the eyes seem to act as keys to open up the doors to these libraries, thus accessing the specific information needed. The particular scanning pattern of the eyes reveals the entire sequence of one's internal strategy for accessing information.

Figure 8 illustrates the direction in which "normally organized" right-handed people will move their eyes in order to access certain types of information (it would be reversed for left-handers). Individuals will move their eyes up and to the right in order to mentally construct brand new visual images, and up and to the left to access previously seen visual images. A similar pattern is seen when people access *auditorily remembered* information (people will look to their left) and *auditorily constructed* information (people will look to their right). The access of *kinesthetic feelings*, including smell and taste, will usually be preceded by people looking down and to their right. This may explain why people will usually look in a particular direction prior to answering questions. The type of information they are trying to access will determine in which direction their eyes will look.

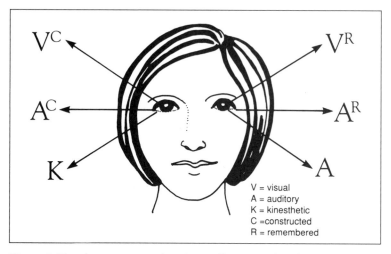

Figure 8. *Visual accessing cues for a "normally organized" right-handed person.*

Consider asking right-handed people the following questions, and notice their eye movements prior to their responses: (1) What color is your bicycle? (visually remembered); (2) How would your mother look with bright purple hair? (visually constructed); (3) What's your favorite current song? (auditorily remembered); (4) What does rabbit fur feel like? (kinesthetic feelings).

It is now known that those nerves that regulate eye movements work very closely with the portion of the brain that governs consciousness by acting as sensory filters. Based on this information, a model of communication has been developed that describes how certain eye movements can be utilized therapeutically to both input important information to the brain and access the information once it is stored. This technology is presently being used as an adjunct to treating physical illness, as a support during emotional processing, and for teaching the art of communication.

LIGHT: FOOD FOR OUR BODIES

Now that we have looked at the relationship of our eyes to our health and well-being, let us look at how our eyes use their basic nutritional food: *light*. Since vision is truly our navigational system, taking in more information per unit of time and from a broader area of space than any of our other senses, it would be useful to examine how our eyes use light to accomplish this task.

As mentioned earlier, each eye contains 137 million photoreceptors.[7] There are approximately 130 million photoreceptors called *rods* and 7 million called *cones*. Cones, which function primarily in the daylight, are concerned with visual acuity and color discrimination at high intensities of illumination; rods, which function primarily in twilight, are mostly concerned with colorless vision and movement at low levels of illumination.[8] These photoreceptors transform light into electrical impulses that are then sent to the brain at approximately 234 miles per hour.[9] These impulses travel along several different routes that involve the entire brain. *Some travel to the visual cortex for the construction of images, while others travel to the brain's hypothalamus* and affect our vital functions.[10]

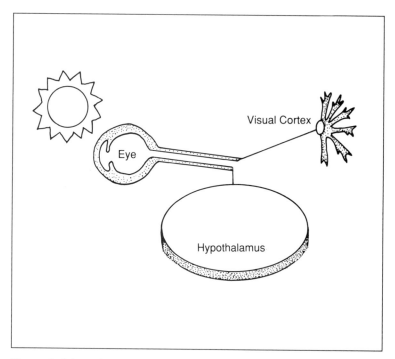

Figure 9. *Major functions of the eyes.*

Although vision is perhaps our most dynamic process, constantly changing in accordance with our mental and physical states, most of us, including scientists and health-care practitioners, think of the eyes as having only a single function: eyesight. Most of us are not aware that *eyesight is merely a small aspect of that dynamic process known as vision.* We are much less aware that our eyes, as the major access routes by which light enters the body, can be mirrors of our general and emotional health as well as accurate indicators of our styles of thinking and learning. This is extremely important inasmuch as this ancient, yet newly discovered, connection between the eyes and the core of the brain functions as the link that bonds us with nature.

This neurological connection was hypothesized in the late 1800s and empirically observed from the 1920s through the 1950s.[11-17] However, it wasn't until the early 1970s that science was able to prove definitively that light entering the eyes was not just for the purpose of vision but was also being sent to one of the most important parts of the brain, the hypothalamus.[18-20] Thus, science established that light entering the eyes serves both visual and nonvisual functions. This discovery proved scientifically what ancient civilizations apparently already knew about light, namely, its route of entry into the body and some of its major effects on the body's regulatory centers and their functions. Did these ancient cultures understand the power of light instinctively, or was their technology and understanding of life far beyond ours?

Consider the ancient Egyptians. Although their technology and achievements remain a mystery to our modern logical minds, they are the same people who utilized elaborately fashioned temples of light to treat the afflicted.[21] The Greeks not only believed in the curative properties of light but specifically thought that light treatments were most effective by way of the eyes. They believed that the eyes were the most accessible path to the internal organs. How could it be possible, therefore, that these ancient cultures, whose technologies still baffle scientists of today, were not aware of these neurological connections? Perhaps the future will reveal to us a third function of the eyes: the ability to bring in the light of consciousness.

When we speak about health, balance, and physiological regulation, we are referring to the functions of the body's major health keepers: the nervous system and the endocrine system. These major control centers of the body are *directly stimulated and regulated by light*, to an extent far beyond what modern science, until recently, has been willing to accept.

THE SYSTEMS THAT KEEP
OUR BODIES IN BALANCE

The central nervous system regulates rapidly changing activities such as skeletal movements, smooth muscle contractions, and many glandular secretions. That portion of the central nervous system that controls and regulates internal functions of the body is called the autonomic (or automatic) nervous system (ANS). It stimulates all of the smooth muscle tissues, the heart, and the glands.

The ANS regulates the inner workings of the body in ways that tend to maintain or quickly restore balance. It does this through two major subsystems, called the "sympathetic" nervous system and the "parasympathetic" nervous system. The sympathetic nervous system supports the body during times of action and movement, while the parasympathetic aids in rebuilding and rejuvenating. You might say that the parasympathetic acts as the engine of the system, while the sympathetic functions as the accelerator and brakes.

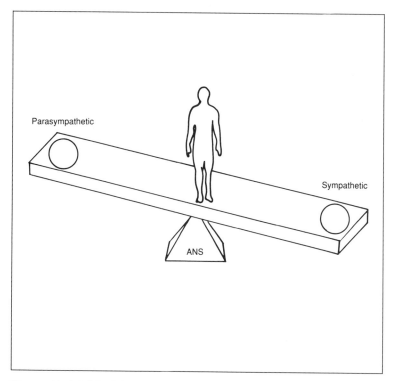

Figure 10. *Model of the autonomic nervous system.*

In general, most of our internal organs are affected by both the sympathetic and parasympathetic nervous systems. If sympathetic signals tend to stimulate an organ, parasympathetic signals tend to inhibit it and vice versa. Thus, our sympathetic and parasympathetic systems together act like an overall system of checks and balances within the entire governmental system of our bodies.

Some of our organs are continually receiving stimulation from both sympathetic and parasympathetic systems, with the dominant of these two opposing influences determining the net effect. For example, continuous sympathetic impulses (e.g., vigorous exercise, frightening experiences, etc.) to the heart tend to accelerate the heart rate, while continuous parasympathetic impulses (e.g., meditation, rest, etc.) tend to slow it down. The actual heart rate is determined by whichever influence dominates. During times of excessive excitement or exertion, the sympathetic nervous system overrides the parasympathetic. On the other hand, the parasympathetic nervous system overrides the sympathetic during conditions of calm, contentment, and relaxation, and in general works to restore normalcy when conditions of stress have been removed.

Although the body's state of balance is constantly regulated by the autonomic nervous system, the ANS itself is merely carrying out the orders of that very important part of the brain, the *hypothalamus*. The hypothalamus, which receives light energy by way of our eyes, *coordinates and regulates most of our life-sustaining functions* and also initiates and directs our reactions and adaptations to stress. It acts like a chief executive officer, passing on orders from the brain (the board of directors) to the rest of the body (the staff) and seeing to it that they are carried out.

The hypothalamus is composed of two major zones.[22] One zone controls the sympathetic nervous system and stimulates hormone production, while the other zone controls the parasympathetic nervous system and inhibits hormone production. As the body's major collecting center for information concerned with its well-being, the hypothalamus receives all external information picked up by our sense organs and all internal signals from the autonomic nervous system as well as the psyche. It functions like the central train station of a large city, receiving the incoming trains with their variety of goods and redirecting them based on the needs of the city and its inhabitants. Its major functions include control of the autonomic nervous system, energy balance, fluid balance, heat regulation, activity and sleep, circulation and breathing, growth and maturation, reproduction, and emotional balance. *Thus, the hypothalamus may be the single most important unit of the brain, standing as high command in maintaining harmony within the body.*[23]

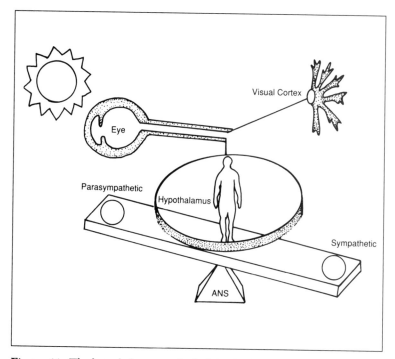

Figure 11. *The hypothalamus as the body's chief executive officer.*

Information received by the hypothalamus is also used to control the secretions of the pituitary gland, thereby significantly affecting the body's other major regulatory system, the endocrine system. In general, the endocrine system regulates the physical and chemical processes involved in the overall maintenance of life (metabolism), as well as the varying rates of chemical reactions within each of our cells. It does this by secreting chemical messengers called hormones directly into the blood stream. Once in the blood stream, these chemical messengers circulate to all parts of the body and affect certain specific target cells that are capable of decoding their messages.

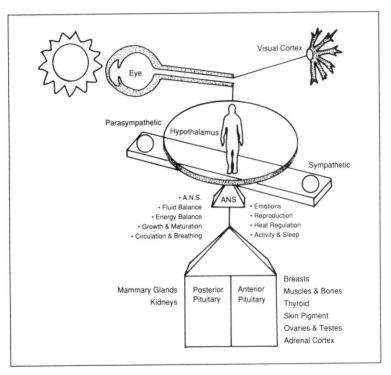

Figure 12. *ANS model with endocrine system.*

The endocrine system consists of the following glands: pituitary, pineal, thyroid, parathyroid, thymus, adrenals, pancreas and gonads. The major gland is the pituitary, referred to as the "master gland" because it controls most of the body's hormone secretions, measuring their amounts as well as making constant readjustments in relation to the body's needs. The pituitary is divided into two distinct portions: the *anterior pituitary*, which affects the thyroid, adrenal cortex, testes, ovaries, breasts, and the growth of long bones, muscles, and internal organs; and the *posterior pituitary*, which affects the mammary glands and kidneys. Although the pituitary plays a key role in the functioning of the endocrine system, it cannot on its own decide the appropriate hormones, or their necessary levels, for specific situations in which the body finds itself. These high-level decisions regarding almost all pituitary secretions are made by the hypothalamus and conveniently sent to the pituitary by way of a direct anatomical connection.

Now that definite anatomical connections between light, the eyes, the hypothalamus, the autonomic nervous system, and the endocrine system have been established, it is important to understand the purpose of these connections. Shakespeare spoke of the eyes as the "windows of the soul." Now it is important to see where those windows lead us.

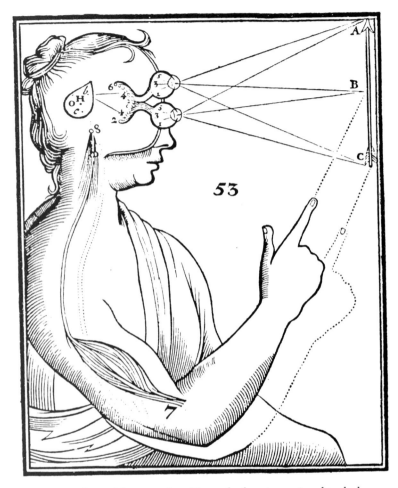

Figure 13. *"Seat of the rational soul" was the function assigned to the human pineal (H) by René Descartes in his mechanistic theory of perception. According to Descartes, the eyes perceived the events of the real world and transmitted what they saw to the pineal by way of "strings" in the brain. The pineal responded by allowing animal humors to pass down hollow tubes to the muscles, where they produced the appropriate responses. The size of the pineal has been exaggerated in this wood engraving, which first appeared in 1677. Reprinted with permission of Richard J. Wurtman, M.D., from an article by Dr. Richard J. Wurtman and Dr. Julius Axelrod,* Scientific American, *July 1965.*

3

The Pineal:
"Seat of the Soul"
— RENÉ DESCARTES

All of life is based on relationship. This begins at conception, when two individuals bond in the process of bringing forth a third. In the womb, the evolving being continues to develop a bond with its mother, which when reestablished at birth becomes the basis for how the child relates with others as well as with the rest of the world. This bond, thought to develop out of the "heart-to-heart" synchronization between mother and child, is a microcosm of humanity's synchronized relationship with nature and the rest of the universe.

The pineal, whose function was *intuitively* recognized by ancient civilizations and, until recently, greatly underestimated by modern science, *serves to assist us in bonding with the universe*. Although it has been variously described as the "sphincter of thought" by Herophilus in the fourth century,[1] as the "seat of the soul" by René Descartes in the seventeenth century,[2] and as the "third eye" by Indian mystics and yogic practitioners, the pineal's functional significance has always been questioned by the scientific world. Earlier in this century it was described as a vestigial structure—an appendix of the brain—having no real purpose. More recently, however, scientific literature has provided a wealth of knowledge indicating that the pineal may, in fact, have a rightful place at center stage as another master gland (in addition to the pituitary) in the body. Thus, this previously discredited portion of the brain *may very well be the newest treasure in science*.

THE BODY'S LIGHT METER

Shaped like a pinecone (and hence its name), the pineal gland is located deep in the center of the brain between the two hemispheres and behind and above the pituitary gland. In humans, it can be located by pointing both index fingers directly behind the ears toward the skull. The point where the fingers would meet, if they could touch, is the approximate location of the pineal. Although it is only the size of a pea, its functions are vast. It acts as the body's light meter, receiving light-activated information from the eyes (by way of the hypothalamus) and then sending out hormonal messages that have a profound effect on the mind and body. Its activity, *regulated by environmental light changes* and the Earth's electromagnetic field, is to transmit information to the body pertaining to the length of daylight.[3] Since the length of daylight is a function of season, this transmitted information from the pineal tells every part of the body whether it is light or dark, whether the days are getting longer or shorter, and what season of the year it is.[4] In this way, our bodies stay closely attuned to nature and are thereby able to make appropriate physiological adjustments that will prepare them for upcoming environmental changes. An example of such an adjustment in the rest of the animal kingdom is the thickening of an animal's coat prior to winter. The animal's body obviously cannot wait for the first snowfall to be reminded that it is time to put on its overcoat.

This system of responding to light is very important, inasmuch as animals in their natural environments breed on a seasonal basis and therefore need to have their bodily functions closely synchronized with nature. The degree of this synchronization, however, is directly related to where the animals live. For instance, animals living at or near the equator experience fewer variations in seasonal synchronizations than those living at the extremes of latitude, where harsh environmental conditions and food shortages necessitate a closer connection with seasonal changes in the environment. In the extreme geographical locations, even the slightest lack of harmony between animals and their surroundings would, for example, delay the birth of their young and thus be catastrophic.

The timing of physiological events is very critical to the health and propagation of a species. Since the pineal gland seems to adjust the entire physiology of organisms to their environment, the physical size of this gland seems to vary according to where animals live. Thus, the pineal is relatively small in animals living at or near the equator, whereas its size increases proportionately the further north or south of the equator animals live.

In certain species, such as the elephant seal, the pineal gland at birth occupies 50% of the brain. If the size of the pineal gland is directly related to the degree to which living creatures are in touch with their environment, does the size of the human pineal (pea size) indicate something about the state of our consciousness? Would a change in our consciousness, and a closer connection between us and nature, increase the size of our pineals? Whatever the answer to these questions, respect for nature by *all* living creatures not only is a moral necessity but is definitely crucial to the longevity and quality of all life.

THE THIRD EYE

In creatures such as birds, lizards, and fish, light stimulates the pineal by penetrating directly through the skull. In many reptiles, the pineal has all the photoreceptive elements characteristic of an eye. It is therefore referred to as a "third eye" because, in many creatures, it resembles an eye in both structure and activity. However, in humans, as well as in all hairy creatures, *light stimulates the pineal exclusively by way of our eyes*, therefore making it an integral part of the visual system. The technical name of the pineal is *epiphysis cerebri*, which literally means "top of brain." It is my belief that humans originally also received light stimulation through the top of the head, as is vividly described in many metaphysical and ancient spiritual writings. This indicates that at one point in human evolution, perhaps prior to the development of the brain hemispheres, the pineal may have actually been positioned at the top of the human brain.

THE REGULATOR

Although the pineal is highly active in human beings when we are young and is responsible for preventing the premature onset of puberty and development of sexual functions, its light-activated information is primarily used to orchestrate all the body's functions and synchronize them with the external environment. The pineal accomplishes this by utilizing light-related messages, which it receives from the body's biological clock within the hypothalamus, to determine when to release its very powerful hormone, *melatonin*.

The secretion of melatonin follows a regular daily rhythm. It is released in response to darkness, reaching its highest level in the middle of the night and its lowest level during the day. During its peak release period (2:00 a.m. to 3:00 a.m.), its level can increase tenfold.[5] Once released, melatonin not only directly affects the body's biological clock but, by being secreted directly into the blood, also has a much more widespread effect.[6] Thus, the pineal acts both as a gland, secreting its hormone directly into the blood, and as an organ, by way of its direct pineal-to-brain connections.[7] Melatonin, secreted in response to darkness, can be found everywhere in the body and affects all bodily functions. It has generally been thought that human melatonin levels do not change in response to light below 1,500 to 2,000 lux (one lux equals roughly the light of one candle). Recently, however, Australian researcher Iain McIntyre has found that melatonin levels can change in response to very small amounts of light (200 to 600 lux) if the subjects are exposed to such light for at least one hour.[8] It would appear, then, that *not a single cell in the body can escape the influence of light striking the eyes.* This ability of the pineal to determine whether it is light or dark outside, and thus tell the body when to work and when to rest, allows our biological rhythms to occur smoothly. *We truly are light bodies.*

To date, approximately a hundred bodily functions have been identified as having daily rhythms.[9] Although these rhythms are genetically programmed to complete a cycle approximately every 24 hours, the precision of their schedule, and their ability to function in concert with other bodily rhythms, requires regular exposure to the sun's day/night cycle. Without this solar influence, the many rhythmic functions of the body would resemble an orchestra without a conductor. A graphic example of this is seen in about 15% of individuals considered blind. These individuals, unable to perceive light, cannot receive the environmental cues necessary to direct their pineal. As a result of this, melatonin secretion is abnormal, thereby causing erratic biological rhythms and a myriad of metabolic disorders and hormonal imbalances. Thus, the sun, acting as our solar system's major conductor, truly keeps our internal orchestra functioning in harmony.

In 1979, Dr. Fritz Hollwich wrote perhaps the most comprehensive and profound publication on the influence of light on the human body.[10] An international authority, renowned researcher, author, and retired professor of ophthalmology at the University of Meunster in West Germany, he was the first to demonstrate conclusively that the stimulatory and regulatory effects of light on the human body take place by way of the eyes. From his studies with blind and cataract patients before and after surgery, Dr. Hollwich concluded that if light perception is absent, temporarily disturbed, or markedly reduced, this creates a significant disturbance in physiological and emotional stability.[11]

Today, the pineal is recognized as playing a major role in every aspect of human function. It acts as the "regulator of regulators." Aside from its documented effects on reproductive function, growth, body temperature, blood pressure, motor activity, sleep, tumor growth, mood, and the immune system, it also seems to be a factor in longevity.[12,13]

Recent studies by Swiss researchers Walter Pierpaoli and Georges Maestroni have shown that the addition of the pineal hormone melatonin to the nighttime drinking water of mice dramatically improves their performance, significantly delays or reverses their symptoms of aging (debility, disease, and cosmetic appearance), and increases their lifespan by 20%.[14] Mice given melatonin lived an average of 931 days, while those not receiving melatonin progressively lost weight and lived only an average of 755 days. The researchers felt that aging was not only initiated in the pineal, but that the age-dependent symptoms of growing old may be due to the progressive decline of melatonin synthesis in the pineal. Pierpaoli and Maestroni suggest that melatonin may play a role in reducing stress and controlling stress-related disease.

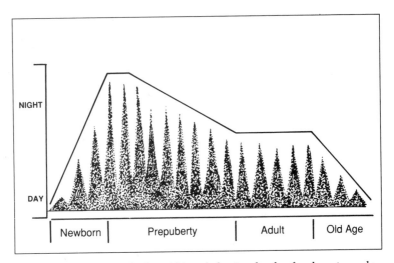

Figure 14. *Melatonin rhythm. Although daytime levels of melatonin tend to be low and constant throughout life, nighttime levels tend to vary substantially with age. Between birth and one year of age, nighttime levels rise significantly, remaining exaggerated until age five. From age five to fifteen nighttime levels gradually drop off, maintaining a fairly uniform rhythm throughout adulthood. In old age (85+ years), the rhythm diminishes greatly.*

In Oriental medicine, the daily patterns of individuals are associated with the level of health they maintain. Imbalanced responses to specific rhythms, seasons, and their associated cycles are related to specific kinds of physical and emotional problems. Harmony within our life processes is related to the level of communion between our bodies and the environment. Can we experience fluid integration of our own minds/bodies/emotions without creating that same level of harmony in our relationships with nature, or vice versa? Isn't our internal integration a mirror of our integration with all life (people, animals, nature, work, etc.)? Perhaps, literally and symbolically, our

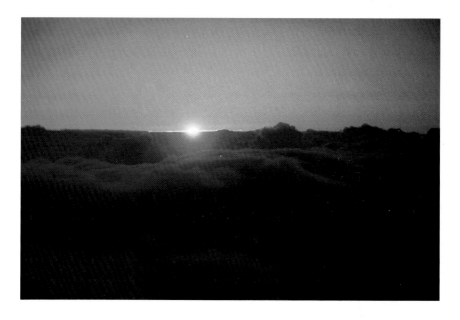

Color plates 1-4. *Sunrise. Reprinted with permission from Laura-Lea Cannon.*

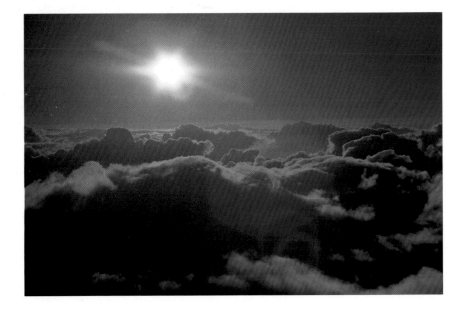

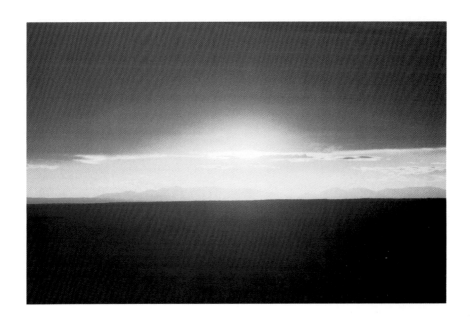

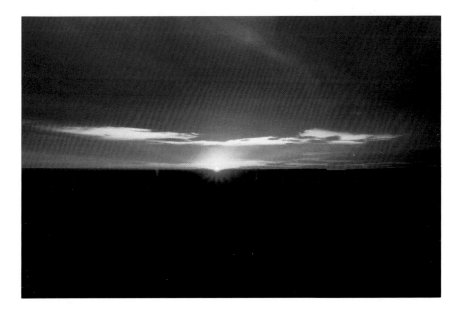

Color plates 5-8. *Sunset. Reprinted with permission from Laura Colan.*

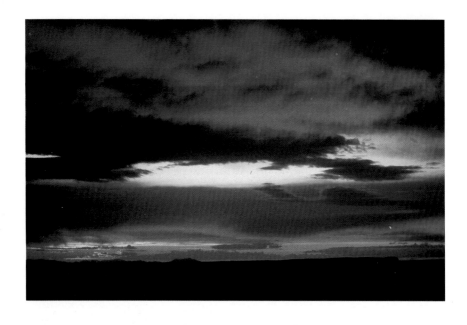

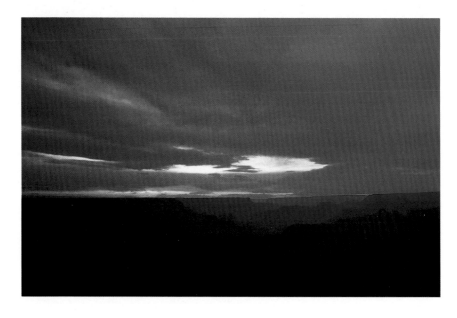

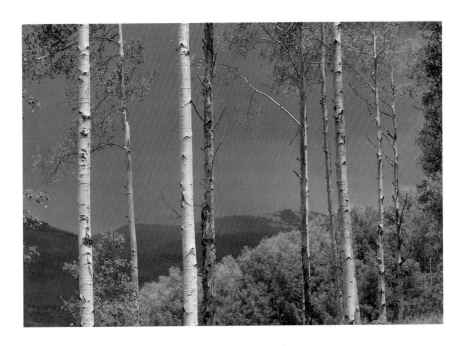

Color plates 9-12. *Seasons. Reprinted with permission from Celia Roberts.*

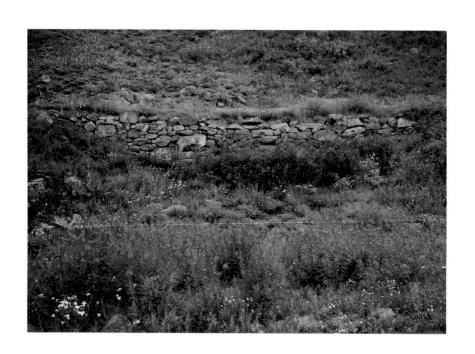

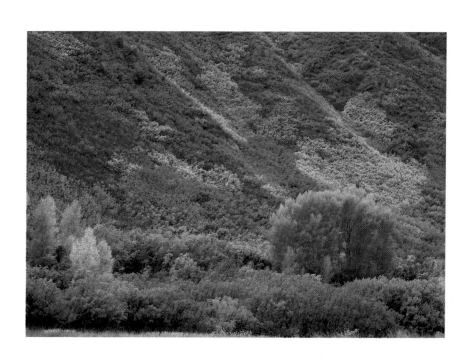

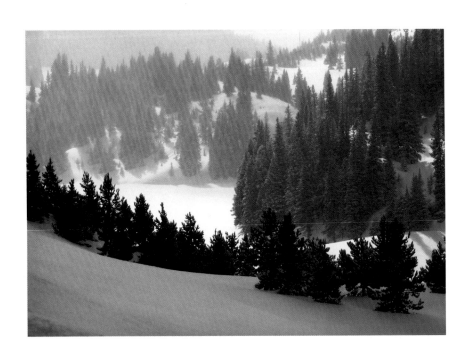

longevity may be related to our ability to integrate and synchronize ourselves with the planetary and solar-stellar energies that surround us.[15] The pineal gland and its interdependence with the rest of the body hold the key to the mysteries of our aging as well as our agelessness.

In summary, light enters the eyes not only to serve vision, but to go directly to the body's biological clock within the hypothalamus. The hypothalamus controls the nervous system and endocrine system, whose combined effects regulate all biological functions in humans. In addition, the hypothalamus controls most of the body's regulatory functions by monitoring light-related information and sending it to the pineal, which then uses this information to cue other organs about light conditions in the environment. In other words, the hypothalamus acts as a puppet master who, quietly and out of sight, controls most of the functions that keep the body in balance.

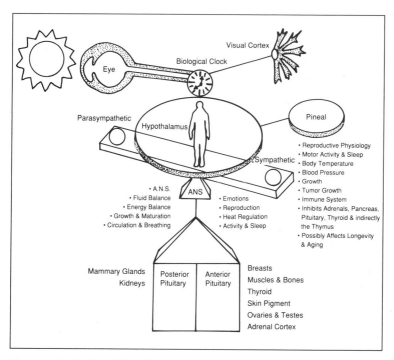

Figure 15. *ANS model with endocrine system and pineal gland.*

All the body's systems relate to each other in a constant state of flux, with the hypothalamus at the center. The hypothalamus interfaces between mind and body, coordinating the readiness of both, affecting our consciousness, and thereby controlling our constant state of preparedness. This critical maintenance of body harmony is effected by synchronizing the body's vital functions with the environmental conditions, or, as some people say, "becoming one with the universe."

4

Color:
The Rainbow
of Life

One evening, my son, Erik, and I were sitting outdoors when he made a profound discovery. Pointing a lit flashlight toward the sky, he said, "Wow, you can't see the light unless it hits something." As I thought about this, it occurred to me that we cannot see anything until light hits it. In other words, light gives life to the objects it strikes, and the objects then appear as colors flowing into forms. Not only do all things appear colored, but our visual perception and discrimination are based initially on color and later on form. Color appears to describe life itself, evoking inner feelings, memories, and responses. It has a power and language of its own, which, when communicated as energy, can excite, sedate, balance, motivate, inspire, enhance learning, and even lure us into buying things we may not need. It vividly describes our states of being in such expressions as "red hot," "feeling blue," "in the pink," "white as a ghost," and "looking at the world through rose-colored glasses." These observations have led me to believe not only that light is responsible for the emergence of all life, but that all life literally is light. Life is truly color-full!

Color, derived from light, is a form of radiation, as are x-rays, ultraviolet rays, and microwaves. The difference lies in the fact that radiation of the wavelengths (or energy) of colored light is visible to us, while radiation of other wavelengths is not. The wavelengths of visible light lie approximately between 400 and 700 nanometers. A nanometer (nm), equivalent to one billionth of a meter, is a standard unit of measurement used to express wavelength. As the wavelength of light gradually increases from 400 to 700 nm, its color, as perceived by human beings, changes from violet through indigo, blue, green, yellow, orange, and finally to red. Although we are affected by radiation of many other wavelengths, we are unable to see it. This is probably due to the fact that we, as humans, evolved under the light of the sun, which reaches the Earth with its greatest strength in wavelengths between 400 and 700 nm. This fact appears to indicate that our interaction with and total response to visible light has been evolving slowly from the beginning of human existence, and now it is deeply ingrained in our nervous systems.

Although science recognizes the effects of x-rays, ultraviolet rays, and microwaves on our physical bodies, there still exists a controversy over whether the visible portion of the spectrum also affects us physically. Visible light differs from x-rays only in its wavelength, so how is it possible that colored light, the portion of the spectrum under which we have evolved and to which we are specifically attuned, cannot be exerting a profound effect on us? The nonvisible portions of the spectrum frequently have deleterious effects on our health. Isn't it possible that the rainbow of visible light that has nourished us since the beginning of time is here to give us life as well as health? (See color plate 13.)

As you look at the world around you, notice that color provides the basic harmony within nature. (See color plates 15-18.) It coordinates, differentiates, and blends all forms of plant, animal, mineral, and human life. Segregating night from day, and altering with the climatic changes of the seasons, color uniquely distinguishes everything in the universe. It acts as a mirror, assisting all of nature's inhabitants to see themselves within the dynamic life processes of other living things and allowing them to act as teachers for each other.

SEASONAL CHANGES

As an example of this, consider the colors of the seasons and their relation to the growth and development of all living things. In the spring of the year, nature awakens and proudly shows off the fresh green so characteristic of youth. Green, the center of the visible spectrum, represents aliveness graced with health and balance. In summer, the second quarter of life, nature warms up and is clothed in the more vibrant colors of the rainbow. Things move a bit more quickly and are occasionally bruised, although this is easily forgotten at this time of year. During the fall of the year, nature enters a magnificent period of accelerated evolution, manifested in its many color changes. Each color change can be likened to a different level of awareness for nature's inhabitants as they enter a different stage of life. In the fall, nature, while parading its colors, manifests its wisdom by preparing for the magical flight that will take it to its next stage of evolution. Leaves, for example, exercise ultimate patience, knowing they will fall in their own time and arrive in the place where they will prepare to begin life again. Winter, stark and cold, clearly exemplifies the extreme black and white aspects of nature. Nature goes inside during this phase and rests, while absorbing energy to begin the seasonal cycle again.

Is this much different from our lives as human beings? We are born in balance and splendor. The first phase of our lives, the "formative years," is the time during which we grow more in size than in depth. In the next phase, as youth still "green behind the ears," we experience many bruises, as exemplified by the old expression "no pain, no gain." We then reach a midpoint in our lives and begin to experience an evolutionary growth spurt not felt in the previous phases. Just as the leaves begin to change in color, showing a change in their receptivity to life, so we often experience major awarenesses in our lives and new levels of "illumination." We begin to experience patience, to understand the secrets of life and living more fully, and to appreciate the miracles within our lives. Finally, the winter of our lives is a time of introspection, when we lay the foundation for future levels of growth and evolution. As we discover the beauty around us, and as we notice that seasonal color changes qualitatively reflect our own life processes, we become aware that color seems to bond us with nature and assist us in recognizing our own beauty.

COLOR, FEELINGS, AND RESPONSES

The theory that color affects our lives was eloquently developed in 1840 by famed philosopher and poet Johann Wolfgang von Goethe. His book on color theory, *Farbenlehre*, was considered the definitive work on the subject until the beginning of the twentieth century.[1] In 1921, Rudolph Steiner, a Goethe scholar and authority on the subject of color, stated in his notebook:

> To live in colour:
> From the colour only the representation spread out in the organism.
> From the representation of colour, feelings.
> From the felt and represented colour, impulse.[2]

Steiner clearly states that colors give rise to the feelings that lead to our actions. Color has always been the thread that weaves us into the fabric of life, for all color is light, and light is life itself.

Color's profound effect on life was probably first recognized by humans when we realized that our existence was dictated by two factors beyond our control: day and night, or light and darkness. All living things are vitalized by the bright reds, oranges, and yellows of daytime, and calmed and rejuvenated by the blues, indigos, and violets of nighttime. The observation of this fact was probably the first realization that the red end of the spectrum is energizing, while the blue end of the spectrum is restorative. Using this information, Egyptian healers prescribed the wearing of certain colors to cure both mental and physical ailments. The well-known Greek philosopher Pythagoras (whose theorems served as the basis for architecture) used color therapy 500 years before the birth of Christ.[3]

As mentioned previously, light entering the eyes serves both visual and nonvisual functions. Light serving nonvisual functions proceeds from the eyes to the older and more centrally located portions of the brain: the hypothalamus, pituitary, and pineal. These very powerful, light-sensitive brain centers probably represent the heart of the brain. Their stimulation immediately affects our physical, emotional, and mental states, to an extent depending on the interpretation and history of the individual. The perception of color arises in two different brain centers. The identification, differentiation, naming, and aesthetic response to color, primarily the result of cultural development and formal education, arises in the more formally educated portion of the brain called the cortex. The more reflexive and instinctive responses to color, which profoundly affect our total organismic functioning, arise out of the more primitive midbrain. This could mean that response to color is deeply set and very much entwined in the entire development of the life process.

Since light plays such a major role in the stimulation and regulation of the body's physiological processes, and since color is merely our perception of light of different wavelengths, is it not logical that different colors might then create different physiological as well as psychological effects on us? The answer to this question becomes obvious when we behold a rainbow, and realize how this miracle of nature affects us emotionally. This would appear to affirm the importance of color and specifically those portions of the spectrum to which the human organism is attuned.

COLOR PREFERENCE

Dr. Max Lüscher investigated the subject of color preference deeply.[4] He found that a person's specific preference for one color and dislike for another color had a definite meaning, reflecting either an existing state of mind, a state of glandular balance, or both. Lüscher believed that people's reactions to color are part of their unique and ancient, primal memory — information coming from deep within their center.

The work of Hill and Marg in 1963 partially demonstrated and verified this hypothesis.[5] Using lights of several different colors, they repeatedly stimulated a specific portion of a rabbit's brain that was an integral part of the pathway involved in the transmission of light information from the eye to the pineal gland. They found that the

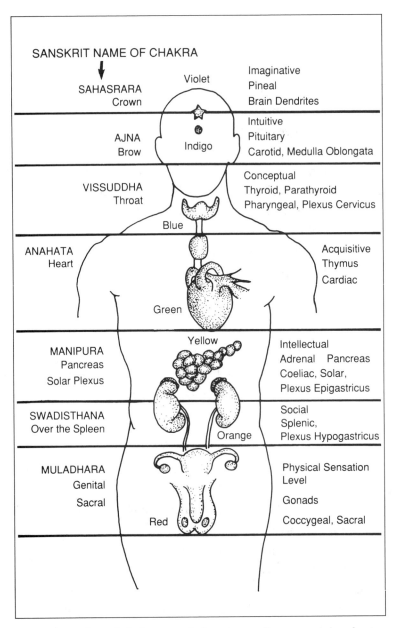

Figure 16. *Etheric link between chakra, personality type, and endocrine secretions. Adapted from a drawing by Christopher Hills, Ph.D. in* Nuclear Evolution; *used with permission.*

rabbit responded differently to each of the different colors.

With the development of more sophisticated diagnostic techniques, science and medicine are continuing to find that certain brain regions are not only light sensitive, but actually respond differently to different wavelengths. It is now believed that different colors (wavelengths) of radiation interact differently with the endocrine system to stimulate or inhibit hormonal production.

Isn't it interesting that, as we enter the 1990s, we are only beginning to scientifically prove knowledge that was intuitively sensed in ancient times? Was it just coincidence that light was originally thought to enter the body through the top of the head and then later thought to enter through the eyes ("the windows of the soul") to the pineal ("the seat of the soul")? Most ancient Sanskrit writings describe the body as having a series of seven major energy centers known as chakras. These chakras, located at the sites of the major endocrine glands and corresponding to particular states of consciousness and personality types, were each responsive to or ignited by a different color. This ancient intuitive knowledge is not much different from the scientific discoveries of the present. Perhaps it is time we realize that our intuitive knowings have preceded our scientific discoveries. *Aren't we in fact using the scientific method to prove what we already know?* Knowledge of the effects of color may prove to be the tip of a most significant iceberg.

In 1942, a Russian scientist, S.V. Krakov, began to examine color vision and its relationship to the autonomic nervous system.[6] By 1951, he had found that the color red stimulated the sympathetic portion of the autonomic nervous system while the color blue stimulated the parasympathetic portion. Krakov's findings were later confirmed in 1958 by Robert Gerard.[7]

PSYCHOPHYSIOLOGICAL EFFECTS OF COLORS

In 1958, for his doctoral dissertation in psychology, Gerard presented one of the most comprehensive studies evaluating the differential effects on psychophysiological functions of viewing colored lights.

His research was designed to investigate and answer the following questions:

1. Does viewing such hues as red or blue arouse different feelings and emotions?

2. If different feelings and emotions are aroused during viewing, are there also correlated changes in autonomic nervous system function, cortical activity, and subjective responses?

In Gerard's study, blue, red, and white lights of equal brightness were each projected separately for ten minutes on a screen in front of 24 normal adult males. The red light increased the viewers' blood pressure, arousal via palmar conductance, respiratory movements, and eye-blink frequency. These same factors decreased under blue or white light. Heart rate showed no appreciable difference under red and blue stimulation. Each color elicited significantly different feelings in the subjects. Blue stimulation increased their sense of relaxation and lessened their anxiety and hostility, while red stimulation definitely increased their tension and excitement. During red stimulation, manifest levels of anxiety significantly correlated with increased physiological activation and subjective disturbance, while the converse was true with blue stimulation. To summarize Gerard's research, the autonomic nervous system and visual cortex (the part of the brain dealing with vision) were significantly less aroused when stimulated by blue or white light than when stimulated by red light.

During that same year (1958), Dr. Harry Wohlfarth also used the autonomic nervous system as a reaction indicator to demonstrate that certain colors have measurable and predictable effects upon humans.[8] According to Wohlfarth's numerous empirical studies, blood pressure, pulse rate, and respiration rate increase maximally under yellow, moderately under orange, and minimally under red, while decreasing maximally under black, moderately under blue, and minimally under green. His findings are illustrated best by the following diagram:

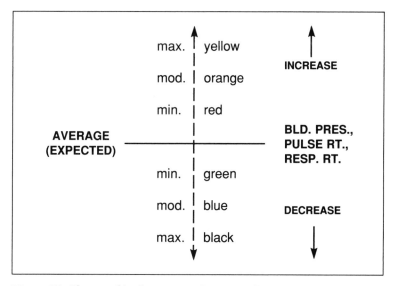

Figure 17. *Change in blood pressure, pulse rate, and respiration rate in response to various colors.*

B.S. Aaronson[9] (1971) and J.J. Plack and J. Schick[10] (1974) also found, as did Gerard and Wohlfarth, that specific colors affect mood, breathing rate, pulse rate, and blood pressure.

BLUE LIGHT FOR JAUNDICE

The use of color as a therapeutic tool now has wide acceptance in both medical and nonmedical applications. The maternity wards of most major hospitals in the country today use blue light (450 nanometers) for the treatment of hyperbilirubinemia (neonatal jaundice). This condition, found in over 60% of prematurely born infants,[11] is the result of a yellow chemical called bilirubin that accumulates in the skin and body tissues, eventually turning the skin yellow. If left untreated, it can cause brain damage or even death.[12] Although it is difficult for an infant to rid itself of this poisonous chemical, it is easily broken up by light, which allows the body to readily eliminate it. The relationship between sunlight and neonatal jaundice was originally noticed in the 1950s,[13] and it was clinically confirmed in 1968 by

Dr. Jerold Lucey at the University of Vermont.[14] He found that when he exposed jaundiced babies to either full-spectrum light or blue light for several days, their bilirubin was lowered to safe levels. Prior to the discovery of light therapy for this condition, the usual treatment was a risky procedure known as *exchange transfusion*.[15] Today, although intense blue light is the most common form of treatment, natural sunlight or full-spectrum light (its close artificial equivalent) have both historically proven to be effective and are, in my opinion, safer and more natural.

Some medical researchers think neonatal jaundice is caused by immaturity of the infants' organs. For example, the liver may not be developed enough to remove toxins from the body. Others think the jaundice is artificially created by a lack of sunlight in modern, windowless nurseries. Since the liver's ability to detoxify the body differs under various lighting conditions, it is questionable whether neonatal jaundice is truly caused by an immature liver or whether it is the direct result of a premature infant's sensitivity to sunlight deprivation. The general lifestyle habits of the infants' parents also need to be considered. In 1900, more than 75% of the United States population worked outdoors, while in 1970 less than 10% did.[16] How much more has the percentage dropped in the last 20 years? By overlooking the importance of natural light in our everyday environment, we may be creating a chronically ill population.

BLUE LIGHT FOR ARTHRITIS

The same blue light found to be successful in the treatment of neonatal jaundice also has been very effective in reducing pain in people with rheumatoid arthritis. In 1982, Dr. Sharon McDonald conducted a study on 60 middle-aged women with rheumatoid arthritis at the San Diego State University School of Nursing.[17] The purpose of the study was to determine the relationship between the degree of pain people experienced and the presence of specific visible wavelengths of light in their environments. Utilizing a simply constructed box with an ordinary incandescent light source shining through a blue filter, Dr. McDonald instructed her subjects to slip their hands into the box through a specifically designed opening while she shined blue light on their hands for varying amounts of time up to fifteen minutes. Although this exposure time was short, a significant degree of pain relief was experienced by most subjects. Based on her results, Dr. McDonald concluded that the reduction in pain felt by these women was directly related to both the blue light *and* the length of exposure. She found that the longer the exposure time, the greater the likelihood of reduced pain. I can personally confirm Dr. McDonald's findings, as I treated my own mother's arthritic hands with a similar filter, with similar results.

RED LIGHT STOPS MIGRAINES

At the opposite end of the spectrum, red light was recently shown to be very effective in the treatment of migraine headaches. In a recent study by Dr. John Anderson, seven migraine sufferers were monitored for up to two years to evaluate the effects of blinking red lights on the severity of their migraines.[18] Using a pair of goggles that alternately blinked red light at different speeds before their eyes, 72% of these patients reported that their severe migraines stopped within one hour of beginning the treatment. Of the remaining 28% (whose migraines did not stop), 93% reported that they felt better. Anderson credited some of the success reported by these patients to their ability to self-adjust the speed and brightness of the lights to a level they found soothing. Most patients found a faster blink rate combined with a higher intensity of light to be most comfortable. When one considers the severe pain and frequent long duration of a typical migraine headache, Anderson's results are quite dramatic.

PUTTING PRISONERS IN THE PINK
AND ATHLETES IN THE RED

Another recent innovation has been the widespread use of *bubblegum-pink* rooms to sedate inmates in prisons across the country.[19-23] When these specially painted, pink holding cells were tested in jails, juvenile reformatories, and other correctional centers, the results were consistently amazing. Some sources reported that a reduction of muscle strength happened in inmates within 2.7 seconds. *Baker-Miller pink* (bubble-gum pink) exerts a physical rather than psychological effect, and it has been proven to calm the most jangled nerves within minutes. Where brute force or sedative drugs were once the only treatment option, small pink holding cells are now used to significantly reduce the incidence of violent and aggressive behavior. Originally spearheaded by clinical psychologist Alexander Schauss of Tacoma, Washington, the use of Baker-Miller pink has now been advocated in hundreds of correctional institutions throughout the world.

Along with the use of blue light for babies, red light for migraines, and pink walls for prisoners, red and blue lights are presently being utilized to improve the performance of athletes.[24] A recent study at a Texas university found that the viewing of red light increased strength 13.5% in viewers and also elicited 5.8% more electrical activity in the arm muscles of viewers compared with other light conditions. This study seems to indicate that briefly looking at a red light may assist athletic performances requiring quick bursts of energy, whereas viewing a blue light may assist in performances requiring a more steady level of energy output. These studies all suggest that specific colors not only affect mood and performance, but also affect commonly evaluated physiological functions. If our moods and vital functions are affected by color, what, then, is occurring on a cellular level?

LIGHT AND CELLULAR CHANGES

One of the most profound and obvious effects of color on a living organism was filmed and described by Dr. John Ott in his movie *Exploring the Spectrum*. While microscopically observing the movement patterns of chloroplasts (cellular components containing chlorophyll) within the cells of Elodea grass, Dr. Ott found that, under full natural sunlight, all the chloroplasts followed a typical streaming pattern of moving around in an orderly fashion inside a cell (figure 18). However, if the observation light was filtered through ordinary glass that cut out

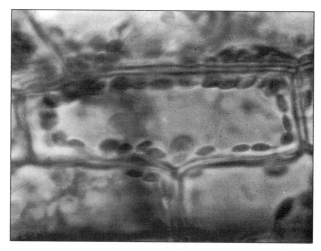

Figure 18. *Chloroplasts under full natural sunlight. Reprinted with permission from* The International Journal of Biosocial Research 7 (1985): 19. *Special subject issue by Dr. John Ott.*

ultraviolet light, or filtered through an ordinary incandescent microscope light source that lacked ultraviolet light, many of the chloroplasts dropped out of their normal streaming pattern and formed a sluggish clump at one end of the cell (figure 19).[25]

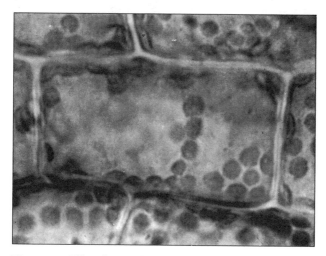

Figure 19. *Chloroplasts under light source lacking ultraviolet light. Reprinted with permission from* The International Journal of Biosocial Research 7 (1985): 19. *Special subject issue by Dr. John Ott.*

Illuminating the chloroplasts through a red filter, which allowed only the longer wavelengths of light through, resulted in some of the chloroplasts remaining in their normal streaming pattern, some totally dropping out of the pattern, and some beginning to short-cut the pattern. If a blue filter was used, allowing only the shorter wavelengths of light through, some of the chloroplasts again remained in their normal pattern, some continued to drop out of their normal pattern, while those that were previously short-cutting moved to a different position prior to beginning their short cut. Dr. Ott also found that when he added some long-wavelength ultraviolet light to the microscope light source, so that it more closely simulated sunlight, *all* the chloroplasts returned to their normal patterns.

By the end of a normal day, chloroplasts, like people, gradually slow down, come to a stop, and then remain motionless during the nighttime period (figure 20). This required period of rest allows them to once again respond to light energy and resume their normal streaming pattern the following day. It appears, therefore, that altering plant cellular function by altering the light source affects the normal process of photosynthesis and the resulting cell chemistry.

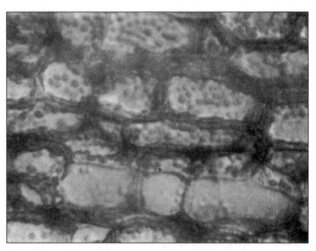

Figure 20. *Chloroplasts at rest. Reprinted with permission from* The International Journal of Biosocial Research 7 (1985): 20. *Special subject issue by Dr. John Ott.*

These cellular effects were again demonstrated in studies conducted at the University of Freiberg in West Germany.[26] The studies vividly illustrated that the wrong kind of light can literally cripple a plant, whereas the right kind of light can allow it to grow normally. (See color plate 14.)

In further studies utilizing pigment epithelial cells from the retina of a rabbit's eye, Dr. Ott found that filtering out normal sunlight also caused abnormal cell function. When he used a blue filter, the cells went through all sorts of contortions, while a red filter caused apparent cell-wall weakening, followed by rupturing and the eventual death of the cell. Is it possible that cellular contortions are the microscopic equivalent of such aberrant human behavior as hyperactivity and anxiety? Could cell-wall weakening be related to breakdowns in the body's immune system? These observations by Dr. Ott clearly demonstrate the life-altering effects of specific wavelengths of light on the cells of plants and animals.

In Dr. Ott's studies, the change in the nature of the cells seem to closely simulate patterns of human behavior. Is it possible that the aspect of human behavior that causes some people to stay in an expected pattern, some to drop out of that pattern, and some to take short cuts through the pattern is related to the light environment in which they live or their biological receptivity to specific portions of the light spectrum? With the amount of time people spend under artificial lighting, which lacks the balanced nutritional aspects of sunlight, it may be possible that some behavioral and physiological differences among humans are in fact partially the result of their relationships to their lighted environment. For example, the habitual wearing of sunglasses could be causing serious problems of which we are not even aware. The subject of artificial lighting and its effects on physiology and behavior obviously needs to be evaluated. By spending an inordinate amount of time under artificial lights, we may be subjecting ourselves to *malillumination*, in much the same way as we subject ourselves to malnutrition by eating an unbalanced diet.

5

Malillumination:
Fact or Fantasy?

Most of us are led to believe that life and learning are difficult and that our goals will be unattainable unless we seek them with a focused mind. We conceive of things as difficult and needing to be sought after, and we therefore frequently also think of them as obscure, complex, and out of reach. Many of us spend our lifetimes chasing mental images rather than observing the realities of life. We constantly wage imaginary wars on nonexistent causes of misunderstood effects and overlook that which is usually right in front of our eyes. When we seek specific things, we frequently miss the important fringe elements in our visual fields; yet those aspects of life that we discover when we're not looking for them are often life's most satisfying.

This general lack of awareness has already led to the toxification of life's most important basic elements: light, air, food, and water. How can things as obvious as these be so disregarded? It is becoming increasingly evident that many human ailments are the direct result of slighting the importance of these elements to our life and health. In recent times, we have become aware that we are constantly ingesting polluted air, devitalized food, and impure water; yet the most obvious nutrient, light, has for the most part been overlooked.

Attempts to deal with air pollution, water pollution, and malnutrition have become major issues within our society. What about *malillumination* (term coined by Dr. John Ott)? Just as an improper diet of foods may cause malnutrition, so an improper "light diet" may cause malillumination, with a similar potential for adverse effects on health. If light is the major nutrient sustaining all life, then it follows that poor and/or incomplete lighting will significantly affect every aspect of human existence. Is malillumination fact or fantasy?

In considering the role light plays in influencing health, it is important to initially look at the constituents of sunlight as well as the kinds of artificial light to which we are exposed in our daily lives. Light is composed of waves of radiant energy. It is measured in wavelengths, the distances between consecutive wave crests. As mentioned earlier, visible light ranges from 400 to 700 nanometers in wavelength. Gamma-rays, x-rays, and ultraviolet rays have wavelengths shorter than 400 nanometers; infrared light, microwaves, and radio waves have wavelengths longer than 700 nanometers. (See color plate 19.) Sunlight, which contains all the different wavelengths, provides the total electromagnetic spectrum under which all life on this planet has evolved. (See color plate 20-A.)

Until 1879, when Edison perfected the light bulb, people spent most of their time outdoors and received adequate daily doses of natural, full-spectrum sunlight. Although Edison's invention was a quantum leap in technology, it simultaneously created a situation in which people lost respect for nature's daily light/dark cycle and began "burning the candle at both ends." With the growing availability of the light bulb, life became largely an "indoor event," which drastically reduced the amount of time to which people exposed themselves to full-spectrum light.

LIGHT IN OUR ENVIRONMENT

The three basic types of artificial light source presently in use are the incandescent, the fluorescent, and the high intensity discharge (HID).

The *incandescent bulb* (similar to Edison's), usually pear-shaped and made to twist into a socket, is most commonly used in today's homes. Its radiant source is a hot filament of tungsten. Although it emits a fairly complete range of the visible color spectrum, it is deficient in the blue end of the spectrum, contains virtually no ultraviolet light, emits much of its light output as yellow and red, and releases its maximum energy as infrared radiation (heat). (See color plate 20-B.)

Fluorescent light sources are the prevalent form of light used in schools, businesses, and industries. Unlike incandescent bulbs, fluorescent lamps generate visible light by nonthermal mechanisms. Fluorescent sources can produce different kinds of light, depending on the phosphors (fluorescent substances) they contain. However, they typically produce a rather distorted spectrum of light, which contains only a limited portion of the total spectrum. The cool-white fluorescent light, the most frequently used, is deficient precisely in those areas of the spectrum (red and blue-violet) where the sun's emission is the strongest. (See color plate 20-C.) The "full-spectrum" fluorescent light, yielding the closest solar match in commercially available lighting, is perhaps the "state of the art" in present-day lighting technology. Its attributes will be more fully discussed later in this chapter. (See color plate 20-D.)

High intensity discharge (HID) lamps, producing a very bright orange-red or blue light, are used mostly outdoors in street lamps and as security lights in high crime areas.

LIGHT AND HUMAN FUNCTIONING

Since most of us spend our waking hours indoors, eliminating sunlight from our daily diets, it is important to discuss this indoor environment in relation to our health, productivity, and general well-being. Perhaps the most comprehensive, yet least known, study on the effects of lighting (and other factors) on human functioning and development was the pioneering work of Dr. Darell Boyd Harmon in "The Coordinated Classroom."[1] Harmon's work began in 1938, when the Texas Department of Health initiated a long-range comprehensive program of child development. This research-based program was instituted as part of the services provided by the school system for protecting and promoting the health of school children.

During the initial phase of this program, a thorough inventory was made to determine any physical and/or psychological problems experienced by the children in the study. Classroom factors that might be related to or contributing to their difficulties were also surveyed. In the first three-year period, over 160,000 school children were screened for health and educational problems, while the physical aspects of over 4,000 of their classrooms were evaluated. Preliminary analysis of this data showed that by the time children graduated from elementary school, over half of them had developed an average of two observable, but preventable, deficiencies. Correlating these deficiencies with classroom factors revealed that many of the difficulties were related to bodily activities aroused when the eyes were stimulated by light. Based on these findings, intensive studies were initiated in 1942 to develop methods for controlling the adverse physical factors in the classroom environment. In 1946, the findings of all the studies were combined and used as a basis for planning an advanced experimental center for the purpose of determining the optimum lighting, seating, and decor to result in maximum school performance with minimal effort. Appropriate changes were then instituted in one of the schools, and a six-month experimental study was undertaken.

Selected health problems revealed at the beginning of the six-month study were evaluated again at the end of the study. There were substantial reductions in several of the children's problem areas, as shown below:

Problem Areas	Percent Reduction
Visual difficulties	65
Nutritional problems	47.8
Chronic infections	43.3
Postural problems	25.6
Chronic fatigue	55.6

In addition to these apparent improvements in physical well-being, some comparable results also were seen in academic achievement, *even though no attempt was ever made in any of the centers to study or augment curriculum, educational philosophy, or methodology.* Harmon's study is of great significance in that it concerned itself with the frequently overlooked organic needs of children in learning situations. Most research instead considers curriculum needs of prime importance. Harmon's study significantly demonstrated the relationship between the classroom environment and health and learning capabilities, although its attention to light was more related to light distribution than it was to the quality of light distributed.

FULL-SPECTRUM LIGHT:
THE WORK OF JOHN OTT

When we speak about the quality of light and its importance to the well-being of all living organisms, the contributions of Dr. John Ott stand out above those of other researchers in the field. Ott, a banker by profession, turned his lifelong interest in time-lapse photography into a full-time investigation of the ecology of light. His pioneering work on the effects that different light sources have on plants, animals, and humans may prove to contain some of the most important discoveries of the century.

While doing some time-lapse photography for Walt Disney, Ott observed that pumpkin seed sprouts would not fully mature under fluorescent lights, but that they flourished if ultraviolet light was added to the light source.[2] Following years of study of the effects of different light sources on plants, he turned his attention to the question of their effects on animals. Some of his earliest studies during the 1950s and 1960s involved measuring the life span of laboratory animals kept under various fluorescent lights as compared to those living under natural unfiltered daylight. His carefully designed and controlled studies, simultaneously undertaken at several top medical schools and research hospitals, consistently demonstrated dramatic differences in the life spans of the experimental animals. For example, mice living under pink fluorescents or daylight-white fluorescents lived an average of 7.5 and 8.2 months respectively, whereas those living under natural unfiltered daylight were much healthier and lived an average of 16.1 months.[3]

Based on the results of these and other studies, Ott concluded that natural light is as important to the life and health of animals as it is to plants. He then recommended to Duro-Test Corporation that it modify one of its fluorescent tubes to more closely replicate the full spectrum of natural sunlight. He suggested that they do this by adding a phosphor that would produce the three types of ultraviolet radiation in the same proportions as they are present in sunlight. Through the investigations, suggestions, and inspiration of Ott, Duro-Test succeeded in developing the first full-spectrum fluorescent tube, the Vita-Lite.

THE EFFECT OF FULL-SPECTRUM LIGHT ON HUMANS

The development of full-spectrum artificial lighting, a significant step in the right direction, prompted Ott to further investigate the possible negative effects of improper lighting on the health and performance of human beings. In 1973, Ott and the Environmental Health and Light Research Institute undertook a study involving four first-grade classrooms in Sarasota, Florida. Full-spectrum, radiation-shielded fluorescent light fixtures were installed in two of the windowless classrooms, while standard cool-white fluorescent fixtures were installed in two other identical windowless classrooms that served as controls. Concealed time-lapse cameras took random sequences of students and teachers in the classrooms. Although teachers were aware of the program, neither they nor their students were aware of when they were being photographed. The photographed results were significant. Under the cool-white fluorescent lighting, some students demonstrated hyperactivity, fatigue, irritability, and attentional deficits. In the classrooms with full-spectrum lighting, however, behavior and classroom performance, as well as overall academic achievement, improved markedly within one month after the new lights were installed. Furthermore, several learning-disabled children with extreme hyperactivity problems miraculously calmed down and seemed to overcome some of their learning and reading problems while in classrooms with full-spectrum lighting.

This study additionally demonstrated that children in rooms with full-spectrum lighting developed *one-third the number of cavities in their teeth as children in the classrooms with the standard cool-white fluorescent lights.* Similar results on the development of cavities were reported by Sharon, Feller and Burney.[4] They found that golden hamsters, raised for a period of fifteen weeks under cool-white fluorescent lighting and fed a cavity-producing diet, developed five times as many dental caries as hamsters raised for the same period of time and with identical diets but under full-spectrum fluorescent lighting. Further, the severity of the decay was ten times greater under the cool-white lights than under the full-spectrum lights. These findings are not surprising, as research conducted in the 1930s on a large number of children showed that the incidence of dental cavities was much higher during the school year (winter, spring) than during the summer months. Also, the number of cavities developed was directly related to the amount of sunlight available in the area where the children lived.[5,6] The more sunlight, the less cavities.

THE EFFECT OF FULL-SPECTRUM LIGHT ON CHOLESTEROL

Recently the poultry industry has been looking at the effects of raising chickens under full-spectrum lighting.[7] Initial reports indicate that chickens raised under full-spectrum lighting do much better than their counterparts living under other forms of artificial lighting. They live twice as long, lay more eggs, are calmer and less aggressive, and produce eggs that are approximately 25% lower in cholesterol.[8] The fact that the eggs laid by chickens living under full-spectrum lighting are lower in cholesterol is not so unusual, considering that human cholesterol levels also drop under the influence of sunlight. Could the problems caused by high cholesterol levels in humans be significantly reduced if farm animals caged in today's typical factory farms, where they never see "the light of day," were reared outdoors under natural sunlight?

What would happen to our cholesterol levels, as well as our general health, if we spent more time outdoors and used full-spectrum light indoors? It is now known that moderate exposure to sunshine affects cholesterol metabolism in such a way that blood cholesterol levels are rapidly and significantly reduced.[9] This information becomes very important when we recognize that approximately 50% of the deaths in this country are attributable to diseases of the heart and circulatory system, which are frequently caused by excessive cholesterol.[10]

FULL VERSUS
INCOMPLETE SPECTRUM LIGHTING

In 1980, Dr. Fritz Hollwich conducted a study comparing the effects of sitting under strong artificial cool-white (non–full-spectrum) illumination versus the effects of sitting under strong artificial illumination that simulates sunlight (full-spectrum).[11] Using changes in the endocrine system to evaluate these effects, he found stresslike levels of ACTH and cortisol (the stress hormones) in individuals sitting under the cool-white tubes. These changes were totally absent in the individuals sitting under the sunlight-simulating tubes. The significance of Hollwich's findings becomes clear when the functions of ACTH and cortisol are examined. Both of these metabolic hormones play major roles in the functioning of the entire body and are very much related to stress response. Since their activity increases under stress, and since both of these hormones also function as growth inhibitors, this may account for the observation that persistent stress stunts bodily growth in children. Hollwich's findings clarify and substantiate the observations of Ott and others regarding the agitated physical behavior, fatigue, and reduced mental capabilities of children spending their entire days in school under artificial illumination. He concluded that the degree of biological disturbance and the resulting behavioral maladaptations were directly related to the difference between the *spectral* composition of the artificial source and that of natural light.

Since cool-white fluorescent lamps are especially deficient in the red and blue-violet ends of the spectrum, this may explain why color therapists have historically used a combination of the colors red and blue-violet as an emotional stabilizer. Hollwich's work not only confirms the biological importance of full-spectrum lighting, but it also reconfirms the importance of specific colors by evaluating the effects of their omission from our daily lives. Based on the research of Hollwich and others, the cool-white fluorescent bulb is legally banned in German hospitals and medical facilities.

The results of good research are very impressive. However, there is nothing like personal experience to cause a shift in one's awareness. I recently received an account of such an experience:

In the middle '70s, during the energy crisis brought on by the oil "shortages," I was working for the state Department of Employment as an employment counselor. Word came down from the state capitol to all managers that electricity was to be conserved by shutting off alternate banks of overhead fluorescent lights. At first the relative dimness seemed depressing, but I noticed that almost immediately the sound level had diminished: we all seemed to speak in lower, more modulated voices. The applicants who sometimes had to sit and wait to be interviewed, whether for unemployment insurance eligibility or job possibilities, also seemed to have less hostility toward us when we finally got to them, and the noise level from the waiting room had decreased. At the day's end, I for one felt much less tired. I remember speaking to some of my colleagues, who also felt the difference, except that they objected to the "gray lights." I mentioned the welcome change to our manager and suggested that perhaps we could function more efficiently with less glaring fluorescents overhead on a permanent basis, and even recommended that he report this to the powers in the state capitol. I was told not to rock the boat, and as soon as the "crisis" was over, the lights came back on, and so did the noise level, the angry voices, and that tired feeling by the middle of the day.[12]

More recently, it has been found that full-spectrum lighting in the work place creates significantly lower stress on the nervous system than standard cool-white fluorescent lighting and reduces the number of absences due to illness. These findings seem to indicate that full-spectrum lighting may act to boost the immune system in the same way as natural sunlight.

USING LIGHT TO REVITALIZE
FOOD AND WATER

If full-spectrum lighting has such positive effects on the body, what are its effects on other basic elements of life, like water and food? Orie Bachechi, of Albuquerque, New Mexico, has been asking this question for many years. He has developed a very interesting product, the Kiva Light, which utilizes a modified full-spectrum light source to revitalize food and water.[13] Bachechi claims that his Kiva Light, placed over water, structures the water so that it is the same as water found around membranes of healthy body cells. He states that water found in cancer cells or other unhealthy cells is not structured in the same way. He also says that the process of structuring not only balances the pH of the water, based on the minerals within it, but it also alters its freezing and boiling characteristics and noticeably changes its taste as well as the taste of foods cooked in it. Bachechi recommends that all foods be prepared under Kiva Lights. He has found that these lights have a profound "energizing and balancing" effect on food, which is transferred to those consuming it. If it is true that the Kiva Light favorably structures water so that it resembles the water around healthy body cells, what happens to the structure of body water in those who spend most of their day under light sources significantly different from sunlight? Could this be contributing to ill health? Although I haven't personally used Bachechi's Kiva Lights, my own experience with full-spectrum lighting and food has yielded similar results. (See appendix A: Full-Spectrum Light Sources and Other Related Products.)

If the absence or imbalance of certain naturally present spectral-light components causes a reduction in our physiological, emotional, and intellectual functioning, then these components of light must play an integral role in the proper biological functioning of all living organisms. As we continue to discover and understand the role that light plays in our lives, its use as both a therapeutic and preventive tool will become more evident. Treatments for conditions ranging from cancer and depression to jet lag and life extension will become common occurrences. History abounds with observations and scientific validation for the health-giving properties of light. From its proven effects on plants to its stimulatory and regulatory effects on the highest neurological centers of human beings, light has taken center stage as the primal element of life. We are now entering the era of "The New Medicine."

PART TWO

Light:
The New
Medicine

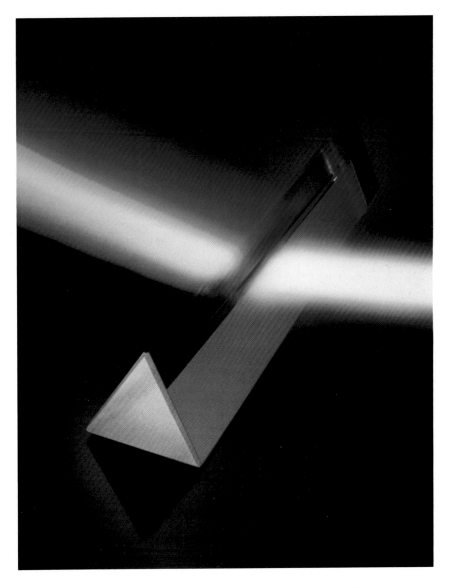

Color plate 13. *Prism. Reprinted with permission from General Electric Corporation, Lighting Division.*

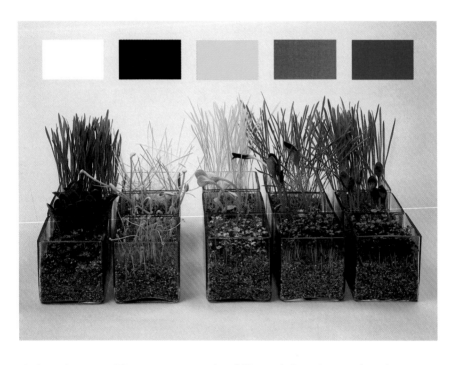

Color plate 14. *Plants growing under different lights. Reprinted with permission from Horst Munzig.*

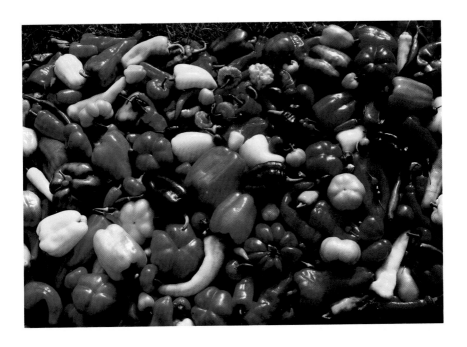

Color plate 15. *Peppers. Reprinted with permission from D. Cavagnaro.*

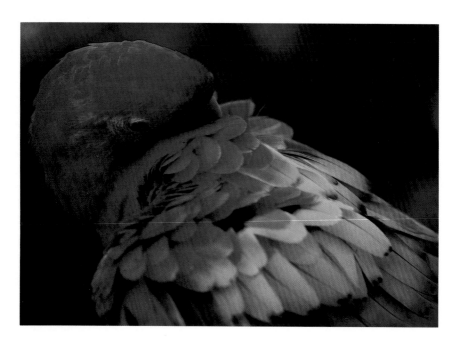

Color plate 16. *Scarlet macaw. Reprinted with permission from Gerry Ellis.*

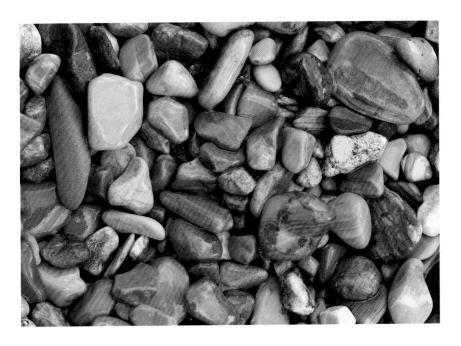

Color plate 17. *Rocks. Reprinted with permission from Charley Gurche.*

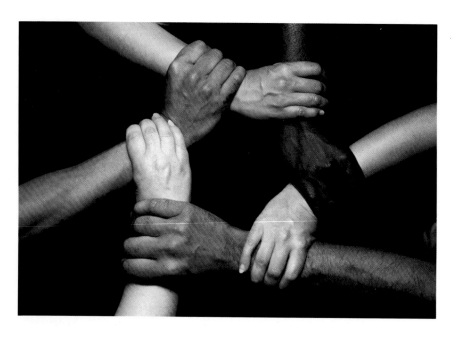

Color plate 18. *Hands. Reprinted with permission from Werner Krutein.*

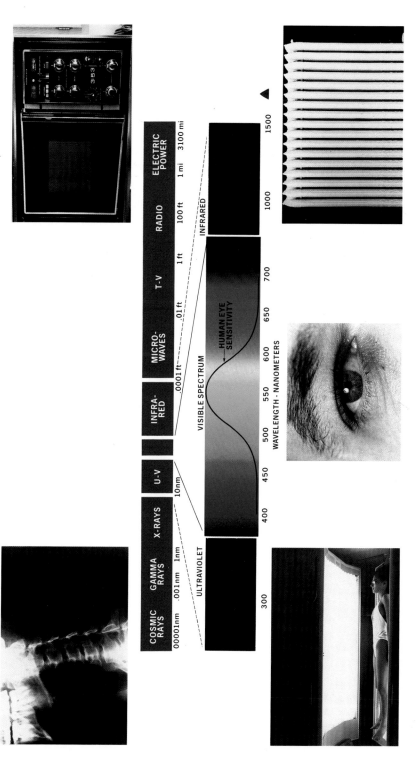

Color plate 19. *Electromagnetic chart. Reprinted with permission from General Electric Corporation, Lighting Division. Peripheral photos by Laura-Lea Cannon.*

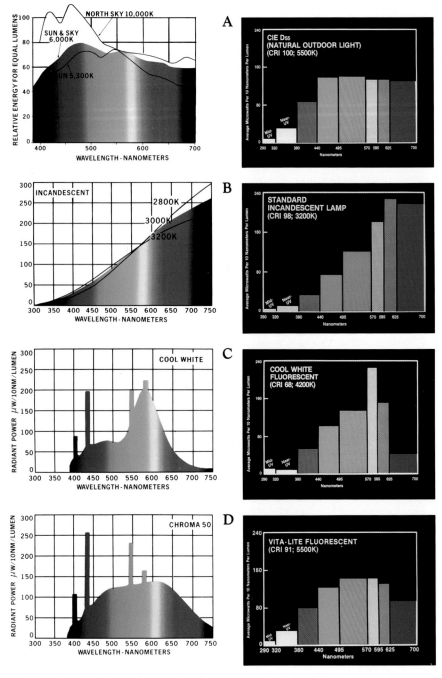

Color plate 20. *Spectral power distribution charts. Left-hand charts reprinted with permission from General Electric Corporation. Right-hand charts reprinted with permission from Duro-Test Corporation.*

6

The Enlightened
Pioneers

It is difficult to say who the real pioneers in the field of light therapy were. Did this work begin with God the Creator saying, "Let there be light," or with Jesus using the light of God to heal people? Light has been with us since the beginning of time. It has been used therapeutically by all the major historical cultures, and it has touched the hearts and creative minds of those who have learned to appreciate its potential. Its physical attributes, scientific properties, therapeutic applications, and relation to the function of all living things have been described by many significant people who have influenced history. Among its earliest medical advocates were Herodotus (the father of heliotherapy), Aurelius Celcus (first-century–A.D. physician and medical writer), Claudius Galen (Greek physician), and Avicanna (Arabian philosopher and physician).[1] These intuitive healers worshiped the sun (light) as a god, recognizing through their own experiences its ability to give, maintain, and restore life.[2]

While early pioneers of light therapy were establishing its medical credibility, others were speculating on light's physical attributes and discovering its scientific properties. For example, Aristotle believed that light traveled in waves, while Euclid postulated that it traveled in straight lines. Claudius Ptolemy, a second-century Alexandria astronomer, noticed that light bends at the boundary between two mediums of dissimilar nature, thus discovering the phenomenon of refraction. In 1672, Sir Isaac Newton, using a prism, was the first to discover that light consists of the colors of the rainbow (the visible spectrum). Then there was Ole Roemer, who in 1676 was the first to measure the speed of light.

Whereas these early physicians and astronomer/physicists worked with and studied the science of light, there were others, such as Hippocrates, Plato, Von Peczely, Shakespeare, and Descartes, who not only saw the importance of light, but also described the eyes as the bridge between the light of God and the spirit of humanity. They clearly recognized that the eyes, illuminating the body, mind, and spirit, represented a gateway into a person's entire being.

However, it wasn't until the 1800s that physicians throughout the world became fully aware of the healing properties of sunlight. At this point in time, cures using light were being claimed for conditions ranging from simple inflammation and paralysis to tuberculosis. Then the 1870s ushered in several significant breakthroughs: practitioners of healing with light, who had primarily used direct sunlight for treatment, began to look at color and its possible rainbow of effects.

General Augustus J. Pleasanton, in 1876, published his book *Blue and Sun-Lights*. He declared that the quality, yield, and size of grapes could be significantly increased if they were grown in a specially designed greenhouse in which panes of blue glass alternated with panes of transparent glass. He also reported curative effects of blue light for both animals and humans. In animals, he found that blue light cured certain diseases, elevated fertility, and increased the rate of physical maturation. In humans, he found blue light to be very effective in treating diseases, especially those accompanied by pain. In connection with a patent granted for his procedures, Pleasanton wrote,

> I have also discovered, by experiment and practice, special and specific efficacy in the use of this combination of the caloric rays of the sun and the electric blue light in stimulating the glands of the body, the nervous system generally, and the secretive organs of man and animals. It, therefore, becomes an important element in the treatment of disease, especially such as have become chronic, or result from derangement of the secretive, perspiratory or glandular func-

tions, as it vitalizes and gives renewed activity and force to the vital currents that keep the health unimpaired, or restores them when disordered or deranged.[3]

In these comments, written more than a hundred years ago, Pleasanton reported using blue light from either the sun or an artificial source as an effective means of stimulating the glands, nervous systems, and secretive organs of both people and animals. He also considered bodies to be living energy systems (as described in Oriental medicine) that are consistently kept in balance by nature's master acupuncturist, *the sun.* Although controversial and scoffed at due to a lack of scientific substantiation, Pleasanton's findings made a significant impact on those who followed him.

The year 1877 not only hosted the discovery that sunlight (specifically the violet end of the spectrum) was very effective in killing bacteria, but also heralded the publication of a new book by Dr. Seth Pancoast called *Blue and Red Lights.*[4] Pancoast, a very prominent physician, used sunlight filtered through panes of red or blue glass to accelerate or relax the nervous system, thus creating balance within the body.

In 1878, Dr. Edwin Babbitt published his classic, *The Principles of Light and Color*, which took the medical profession by surprise.[5] His book was the most credible and outstanding work on light and color of its time. Unlike his predecessors, Babbitt didn't just treat people with sunlight filtered through panes of colored glass, but developed several different devices that combined colored filters with both natural and artificial light. One of his devices, the Chromo Disk, could be fitted with specific filters and then focused on desired areas of the body for treatment. He also developed special solar elixirs by irradiating water with sunlight and then filtering it through a special Chromo Lens. According to Babbitt, this "potentized" water retained the energy of the vital elements within the particular filter used and had remarkable healing powers. Solar tinctures are still manufactured and used today by many color therapists. Unlike Pancoast, who primarily used the red and blue portions of the spectrum for treatment, Babbitt incorporated many different hues, thus broadening his treatment capabilities. Many thought him a miracle worker, as he would frequently treat the most stubborn ailments with success. Though the contributions of Babbitt, like those of Pleasanton and Pancoast, were never fully acknowledged, they did stimulate a new interest in light and color that still lives on today.

During the 1880s and 1890s, many specific bacteria were found to be sensitive to ultraviolet light. These discoveries led to the extensive use of ultraviolet as an anti-bacterial agent for both medical and non-medical purposes. It was used to disinfect hospital and operating rooms, as well as to treat wounds, burns, and respiratory infections.

SUNLIGHT AND VITAMIN D

One of the most important phototherapeutic discoveries of the 1890s was that rickets, a disease characterized by a deformation in the developing bones of young children, could be cured by sunlight. Although the reason for sunlight's effectiveness was not immediately understood, it was later discovered that sunlight striking the skin initiated a series of reactions in the body leading to the production of vitamin D,[6] a necessary ingredient for the absorption of calcium[7] and other minerals from the diet. If vitamin D is absent, the body will not absorb the amount of calcium required for normal growth and development of the bones. This deficiency leads to the condition called rickets in children and osteomalacia in adults, which is characterized by a weak, porous, and malformed skeleton.[8] It is now known that both the development and maintenance of healthy bones is dependent upon the body's ability to absorb calcium and phosphorus.

The vitamin D manufactured by the body in response to sunlight, called vitamin D_3, is not a true vitamin but a hormone called cholecalciferol that is produced by the body in response to ultraviolet radiation. It is different from the commercially produced D_3 found in most dairy products and the vitamin D_2 (ergocalciferol) found in most vitamin tablets and fortified foods. Naturally produced D_3 is more effective in the body and has never been found to be toxic, whereas dietary D_2 can be toxic at high levels. Sunlight is now recognized as being the catalyst for the reactions producing the body's main nontoxic source of vitamin D.

A major light-therapy pioneer of the 1890s was Niels Finsen of Denmark, who noticed that tubercular skin lesions were very common during Norwegian winters but very rare during the summers.[9] Assuming that a lack of sunlight might be the cause of the lesions, he began using a carbon-arc light source in 1892 to treat lupus vulgaris (a tubercular skin condition) and eventually used red light to prevent scar formation from smallpox. Years later, he wrote of the photochemical properties of sunlight and established a light institute for the treatment of tuberculosis. His work was so innovative and effective that in 1903 he was awarded the Nobel Prize for being the first person to successfully treat skin tuberculosis with ultraviolet light. During his many years of work with both sunlight and ultraviolet light, Finsen reported miraculous cures on thousands of patients. He is known as "the father of photobiology."

The nineteenth century came to an end with the discovery of x-rays (1895). By then, seeds planted by many of the century's early pioneers had begun to sprout within the minds of two men who would become instrumental in developing the foundation for the present-day science of phototherapy. These men, Dinshah P. Ghadiali and Dr. Harry Riley Spitler, gave birth to the sciences of Spectro-Chrome and Syntonics, respectively. Having studied the work of Pleasanton, Pancoast, and Babbit, Dinshah (as he was known) and Spitler set out independently to evaluate the validity of their predecessors' theories and applications. Dinshah, having an extensive background in physics, chemistry, mathematics, and electricity, focused on developing a precise scientific approach to the application of color to the human body. Spitler, a trained physician, initially looked at the human physiological response to light and from this developed comprehensive and unique clinical applications that were specific for different body types. Whereas Dinshah's Spectro-Chrome system applied color directly to the body,

Spitler's Syntonic approach treated the body by way of the eyes, thus using the shortest and most direct path to the brain centers.

SPECTRO-CHROME

Dinshah P. Ghadiali, born in India in 1873, first evaluated his forerunners' color theories in the year 1897. He spent the next 23 years thoroughly researching the basis for his healing system. Then in 1920, with his research completed, he founded the Spectro-Chrome Institute and began training both medical and nonmedical practitioners. His three-volume *Spectro-Chrome Metry Encyclopedia* was published in 1933.[10]

Dinshah felt that the science of healing should not use a hit-or-miss approach but should have the exactness and repeatability of mathematics. On this premise, he looked at the basic chemical elements that comprise all living things. Like Babbit, he noticed that every chemical element in an excited state gives off, when viewed in a spectroscope, a characteristic and distinctive set of colored bands called spectral emission lines. This characteristic set of frequency emissions, known as Fraunhofer lines, is the identifying fingerprint for a specific element. Additionally, if an excited element is exposed to white light, it will absorb from that light all the frequencies it had been previously emitting. In other words, all excited elements in the presence of any light will absorb from that light those frequencies that they themselves give off. You might say that light becomes the nutrient for these elements.

Dinshah reasoned that since elements in an excited (live) state *give off* light as well as *absorb* energy from light, it would make sense that the live human body, which uses many of these elements and gives off light by way of its aura, would also absorb light. Based on this reasoning, he studied the Fraunhofer spectrum for each element in the body to determine its predominant color and then matched each element's primary color emission with its known physiological function. He theorized that the major color emitted by an element was related to that element's function in the body; therefore, when used therapeutically, this color would aid the activity of this element in the body.

Combining his extensive research with sound intuition, Dinshah developed a mathematically precise set of twelve attuned color filters to be used with the Spectro-Chrome system of healing. These twelve filters (red, orange, yellow, lemon, green, turquoise, blue, indigo, violet, purple, magenta, and scarlet), enclosed within a projector, were tonated (shined) directly on the desired body parts, as illustrated below. Dinshah used the word *tonation* to mean "the shining of a Spectro-Chrome color on the body."

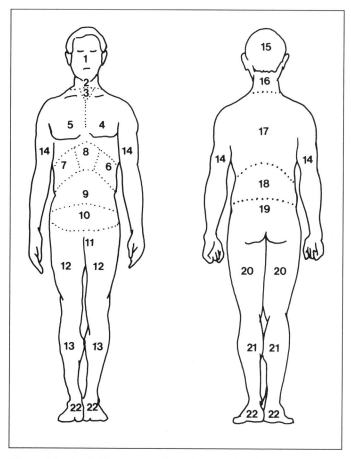

Figure 21. *Dinshah's tonation chart. Reprinted with permission from* Let There Be Light, *by Darius Dinshah.*

After many years of clinical experience, Dinshah recognized a few fundamental patterns that could assist a therapist in determining which colors to use for certain basic conditions. He regarded green as a physical equilibrator and recommended that it, or one of its derivatives (lemon or turquoise), be included in almost all tonations. Lemon (half green, half yellow) he considered to be the "chronic alternative," and he recommended it for all persistent disorders, while turquoise (half green, half blue) he considered the "acute alternative," to be used in all recent (acute) conditions. The use of purple, scarlet, and/or magenta was recommended in all conditions involving the heart, circulatory system, or reproductive system. Purple was used for cases of overactivity, scarlet for underactivity, and magenta for balancing. In all cases of paralysis, the combination of lemon (half green, half yellow) and orange (half red, half yellow) was suggested. In cases of paralysis of the senses, red was added to this regimen. Indigo was utilized in all conditions involving pain, bleeding, and abscess.

Dinshah's theories have not yet been scientifically validated. However, the success of his methods can be verified by all who have used them. Among his most vocal supporters was Dr. Kate Baldwin, senior surgeon for 23 years at Philadelphia Woman's Hospital. Having incorporated the Spectro-Chrome system in both her hospital and private practice, she spoke of its medical value at a clinical meeting of the Pennsylvania Medical Society in 1926. The following is from an abstract of her presentation:

> For about six years I have given close attention to the action of colors in restoring the body functions, and I am perfectly honest in saying that, after nearly thirty-seven years of active hospital and private practice in medicine and surgery, I can produce quicker and more accurate results with colors than with any or all other methods combined — and with less strain on the patient. In many cases, the functions have been restored after the classical remedies have failed. Of course, surgery is necessary in some cases, but the results will be quicker and better if color is used before and after operation. Sprains, bruises and traumata of all sorts respond to color as to no

other treatment. Septic conditions yield, regardless of the specific organism. Cardiac lesions, asthma, hay fever, pneumonia, inflammatory conditions of the eyes, corneal ulcers, glaucoma, and cataracts are relieved by the treatment.[11]

Although Dinshah was not formally trained in medicine, by the time his *Spectro-Chrome Metry Encyclopedia* was published he had been awarded at least four honorary medical degrees.

SYNTONICS

During the same period of time that Dinshah was developing the Spectro-Chrome system, Dr. Harry Riley Spitler was brainstorming an idea that could revolutionize medicine. In 1909, having earned four doctorates and having studied the work of Babbit and others, Spitler began researching and clinically using light therapy in the sanatorium that he directed. He continued using his light-therapy techniques until 1919.[12] Then, clinical observations led him to consider applying these same techniques through the eyes. Because of the highly positive results he achieved with this application, he decided to investigate further the effects of light energy on living organisms.

During 1923 and 1924, Spitler began a series of impressive experiments to evaluate the responses of different groups of rabbits living under different lighted environments.[13] The colors of light under which the rabbits lived were created by means of light filters placed in front of their cages. All other variables (housing, nutrition, etc.) were kept the same for each group. Within three to eighteen months from the onset of the study, some startling results became apparent. The rabbits began to develop abnormal conditions such as loss of fur (some total, some partial), toxic symptoms, abnormal body weight, digestive problems, sterility, abnormal bone development, and cataracts. These conditions must have been related to the different colored lights under which the rabbits were living.

Recognizing that imbalances in both the autonomic nervous system and endocrine system were involved in the development of the abnormalities seen in these rabbits, Spitler further investigated how light might be affecting these systems. His research convinced him that the portions of the brain that directly control both the autonomic nervous system and the endocrine system are also connected to the eyes by the shortest, most direct, and most highly organized nerve pathways in the brain. He concluded that although heredity, environment, and nutrition play major roles in our lives, light may play the most significant role in altering function, behavior, and physiological response; in other words, merely altering the color of light entering the eyes can disturb or restore balance within the autonomic nervous system and thus effect resultant functions.

In 1927, Spitler began developing the first light-dispensing instruments for ocular application.[14] Having both optometric and medical degrees, he recognized that light therapy by way of the eyes could augment the major control centers in the brain that regulate all body functions. Since the functioning of the eyes is directly dependent upon and mediated through the nervous system, this form of treatment could directly affect visual function. Spitler had discovered a "master key" that could open the doors to a whole new healing approach. From discoveries made during his seventeen years of ongoing research, Spitler conceived the principles for a new science that he called "Syntonics."

Syntonics, from the word syntony (to bring into balance), refers physiologically to a balanced, integrated nervous system. Spitler's system of treatment was more comprehensive than that of his predecessors. Not only did he apply light by way of the eyes, he treated people according to their physical/emotional make-up and constitutional type. Realizing that people's general make-up significantly affects their functioning, he created a system based on the premise that not all individuals process and utilize light the same way. He was not concerned with the color of light he was using, but primarily with the power factor, or energy content, of the frequency transmitted by a particular filter. Many different frequencies of light appear similar in terms of their color. Therefore, Spitler assigned a Greek letter designation to each of the filter combinations in order to assist in their differentiation. Although he had approximately 31 different filter combinations in his treatment regimen, only 20 were commonly used.

After extensive research and clinical use had validated the effectiveness of Syntonics as a therapeutic tool, Spitler established the College of Syntonic Optometry in 1933 as a research and educational center for his work. In 1941, he completed his thesis, *The Syntonic Principle*, which then became the definitive text for this new science. The college defined Syntonics as that branch of ocular science dealing with selected portions of the visible spectrum. When its methods are applied by way of the eyes, Syntonics reflexively affects the body's major supportive functions by bringing them into balance with the environment, resulting in improved vision. A post-doctoral educational optometric organization for 58 years, the college offers yearly conferences dealing with the constantly evolving field of ocular phototherapy. (See appendix B: a directory of College of Syntonic Optometry practitioners.)

The discoveries of Dr. Harry Riley Spitler, a researcher a hundred years ahead of his time, scientifically validated that the eyes truly are "the windows of the soul" and opened the door to the emergence of a new "vision" for vision specialists.

7

A New
Vision for
Vision Specialists

The contributions of Babbitt, Finsen, Dinshah, and Spitler established a foundation from which a very powerful nonintrusive science of light therapy could have emerged. However, by the late 1930s, when the College of Syntonic Optometry was just getting off the ground, a turn of events pushed light therapy behind the scenes for many years. Gerhard Domagk, a German biochemist, won the Nobel Prize for successfully treating bacterial infections with sulfanilamide.[1] The discovery of this new "silver bullet" in medicine ushered in an era of pharmacological dominance that paid no homage to the wonderful nonintrusive discoveries of the past hundred years. Light therapy, once considered a miracle cure by many, began to be regarded as witchcraft. Overshadowed by the new wonder drug (sulfa), light therapy became almost obsolete as it went temporarily underground.

It is a shame that we didn't realize back then that our lifestyles, rather than bacteria, were the cause of most diseases. Waging a war against bacteria is like waging a war against ourselves, since many bacteria normally exist in balance within us and only contribute to our disease processes as a result of our own imbalances. For example, under normal conditions, approximately fifteen different kinds of bacteria live within the tear film of the eye; they create no problems for us unless something occurs to create an imbalance in this tear film.

Another way of looking at this is to realize that anything we pay attention to we give life to. It doesn't matter whether the attention is

79

positive or negative. Any type of attention given to something brings it to life, exaggerates its size, and in general acts like fertilizer does for a plant. If a bully picks on someone smaller than himself, sooner or later the smaller person becomes stronger and begins to fight back.

Bacteria, like humans, respond in the same way. In reaction to antibiotics, they become stronger, gradually develop resistance, and finally evolve into new strains that we can't even identify, much less fight against. A powerful illustration of this point is all the resistant strains of bacteria and highly evolved viruses that have developed since Domagk's discovery in 1939. Perhaps, once again, we need to look inside ourselves rather than outside ourselves for the causes of life's ailments.

For the field of light therapy to survive, it became obvious that additional evidence was needed to further substantiate the therapeutic use of light. In 1936, Dr. T.A. Brombach, a noted vision researcher, presented a new finding that would eventually become a major diagnostic and prognostic tool in the field of Syntonics.[2] The results of his research indicated that 69% of children with diagnosed reading problems had a measurable enlargement in the portion of the optic nerve originating in the back of the eye. This condition, usually associated with pathology, is appropriately referred to as an enlargement of the "blind spot" because the portion of the optic nerve affected is functionally a nonseeing area. Although Brombach did not believe that such a condition was pathological, he felt that the presence of this condition could reduce the likelihood of full visual perception and thereby inhibit reading ability.

Further substantiation of Brombach's work came from the conclusions to three published studies by Dr. Thomas Eames, a physician at Boston University. Eames found that

1. Nine percent of the school children in these studies had constricted fields of vision, and of these 9%, 83% were failing in school work in one or more subjects;

2. Visual field constrictions significantly limited the speed of visual perception; and

3. Children with learning disabilities consistently had smaller visual fields than children without learning disabilities.[3-5]

The findings of Brombach and Eames are closely related in that it is now known that a visual field constriction is frequently associated with an enlargement of the "blind spot." Today, both of these conditions are usually linked with pathology of the eye and/or brain, head trauma, high fevers, toxicity, or consequential psychological disturbances. It is significant, therefore, that in the cases of Brombach and Eames these eye conditions were thought to be of functional origin and not related to disease. Eames's findings were probably the visual representation of a more generalized physiological constriction. It is difficult to say whether the academic stress that these children were under caused the visual field constrictions, or vice versa. From my own clinical experience, I have found that, under stress, people have a tendency to constrict physiologically, emotionally, perceptually, and functionally. Additionally, Virginia I. Shipman, in a paper presented to the Eastern Psychological Association, stated that, under stress, an individual's perceptual fields constrict, causing them to "observe less, see less, remember less, learn less, and become generally less efficient."[6]

SEEING SPACE AS A WHOLE, NOT THROUGH A HOLE

To fully appreciate the relevance of these findings, it is imperative to understand the roles our visual fields play in our daily lives. A person's field of vision is his or her ability to simultaneously perceive things peripherally while looking straight ahead. The expanse of this global visual area—left, right, up, down, and straight ahead—is known as the field of vision. Traditionally, the peripheral field of vision functions to perceive movement rather than detail and to dynamically predict how much the eyes will have to move to perceive the next object of interest while they are looking at the present object of regard.

Not only do our fields of vision represent how much of the world our brains are perceiving visually, but more specifically, to me, they represent how much of the brain is actually functioning. The field of vision acts like the root system on a tree. Just as the extent of a tree's roots are directly related to the tree's stability, so the expanses of our fields of vision also act to support our postural, emotional, and physiological stability in the world. If a tree's roots were gradually trimmed closer and closer to its base, its physical stability would gradually be reduced and it would eventually fall over. Humans function in a similar manner. As our visual fields gradually contract due to physical or emotional stress, we perceive less and less and eventually look at the world through a "hole," rather than perceiving it as a "whole."

Recently, this effect of stress on vision was confirmed in a series of studies by Mark Anderson, Ph.D., of Beloit College and Jean Williams, Ph.D., of the University of Arizona.[7] Their studies found that stress directly affects the peripheral field of vision, thus reducing how much we see. They discovered that as the degree of stress increased, so did the likelihood that an individual's field of vision would contract when required to respond to a visually demanding task. They also speculated that coping ability, rest, and diet, if out of balance, could worsen the problem.

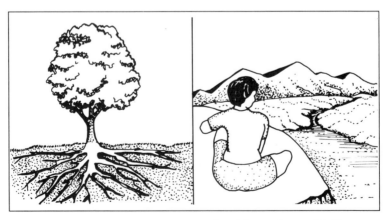

Figure 22. *Tree's root system as compared with human's visual field.*

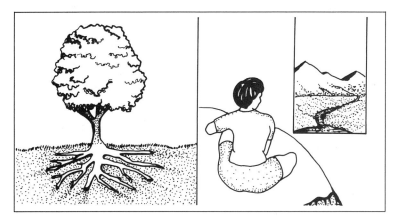

Figure 23. *Trimmed root system as compared with partially constricted visual field.*

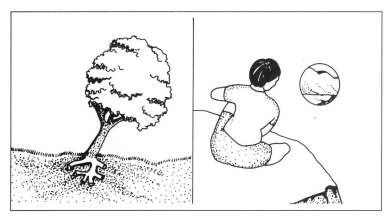

Figure 24. *Loss of stability as a result of extremely limited root system or very constricted visual field.*

The most visually demanding and stressful tasks appear to be school work in general and reading in particular. In the United States, for example, there is an epidemic of poor eyesight. This deteriorization in eyesight usually begins in individuals after they enter school and is rarely seen in cultures where "higher education" (reading) is not stressed. As of 1975, 88% of all postgraduate students in the United

States and approximately 45% of the total United States population were nearsighted! Could this be the reason that both Brombach and Eames reported irregularities in the fields of vision of children with reading and general academic problems? Perhaps stress contracts the visual field, causing a reduction in information processing and resulting in a decrease in learning ability. A 1931 *Popular Science Monthly* article entitled "Noise Causes Bad Eyes" further emphasizes the relationship of stress to visual problems and visual field constrictions:

> City dwellers may not be able to see as well as their country cousins on account of loud street noises. Recent investigations in Russia by Professor P.P. Lazarev and Dr. L. Kuper show that loud noises narrow the field of vision of many persons. This would seem to indicate a reason for the many people found in cities who wear glasses when reading, since they travel to and from their work on roaring subways and elevated trains.[8]

THE CASE OF HARRY

To illustrate how a visual-field loss limits learning capabilities, consider the case of Harry, who at age fourteen and a half was referred to me to evaluate whether his poor vision was contributing to his learning disability. He was nearsighted with astigmatism, had been evaluated as legally blind (20/200) without his glasses, and had suffered from two outbreaks of herpes. My initial evaluation showed no apparent health problems or significant change in prescription, but it did reveal an extremely significant visual-field contraction.

In the test displayed in figure 25, the patient is instructed to look through the visual-field charting instrument at the fixation point (o) located in the middle of the recording chart. The test is administered to one eye at a time. While the patient is looking at the fixation target (o), he or she is asked to say when a white or colored dot moving in from the side toward the middle of the visual field is first noticed. The point of first perception is recorded for all meridians (left, right, up, down, oblique) for both eyes.

To understand this more clearly, attempt it yourself. While looking straight ahead at a target approximately 20 inches in front of you, close one eye and hold both arms out to your sides, thumbs up. Now slowly move both arms towards each other until you first notice each thumb. You will notice that the thumb on the side of your open eye will be seen first. The distance between the two thumbs in degrees equals the horizontal expanse of the field of vision for the eye being tested. You can now repeat the test vertically and obliquely to give you

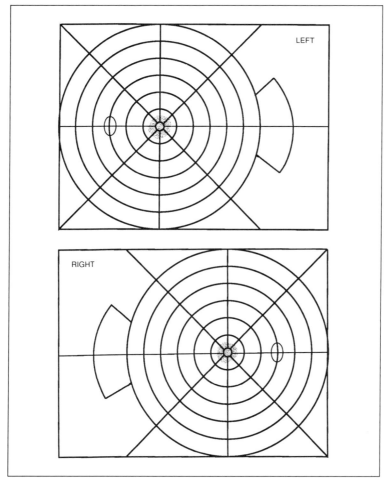

Figure 25. *Harry's visual-field charts prior to treatment. Chart design reprinted with permission from Dr. John Downing.*

the complete visual field parameters for that eye. Repeating the entire test closing the opposite eye will give you a complete measurement for both eyes.

If Harry had conducted this test on himself, he would not have noticed his two thumbs simultaneously until they were *within four to six inches of each other*. How does your field of vision compare to Harry's? Can you imagine how someone perceiving the world through Harry's eyes would feel and respond to everyday tasks like listening, reading, and driving a car?

To understand where we are in any process, we need to know where we've been. Knowing where we are then acts as a foundation for where we are going. Perceiving the world through a small field of vision yields a very limited view of where we've been or where we're going, resulting in a feeling of being lost in space. We become contracted and inward, and thus we perceive less, learn less, remember less, and in general, move with great trepidation. This describes the typical child diagnosed as learning disabled or any human being who is frightened or under emotional stress. Can you personally relate to this description? The sizes of our visual fields are dynamically related to our states of being at any particular point in time, and they literally expand or contract in relation to our consciousness and quality of breathing.

Further evaluation with standardized educational tests revealed that Harry's ability to remember what he saw as well as what he heard was below that of a three-year-old. I recommended that Harry come in five times per week for four weeks in order to receive syntonic treatments (light therapy through the eyes). His daily 20-minute treatment consisted of his looking at a yellow-green light for ten minutes and then a ruby-colored light for ten minutes. One month after the onset of treatment, Harry looked and acted like a different human being. Aside from the dramatic change in his visual field (figure 26), his nearsightedness was reduced by 33%, his eyesight improved to 20/40 without glasses, his auditory memory showed an *eleven-year improvement* (the equivalent of improving one's auditory memory from that of a nine-year-old child to that of a twenty-year-old adult), and his visual memory was now *above that of an eighteen-year-old.*

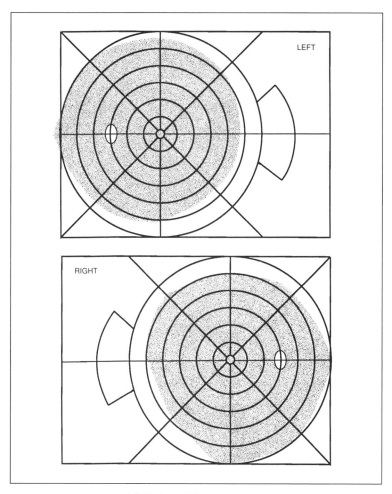

Figure 26. *Harry's visual-field charts following treatment. Chart design reprinted with permission from Dr. John Downing.*

THE NEW VISION THERAPISTS

The discoveries of Brombach, Eames, and others critically changed the clinical direction of Syntonics for optometric vision specialists. These optometric specialists began using visual-field size as a major diagnostic and prognostic tool to evaluate their treatment of functional vision problems affecting learning and general performance. As their clinical experience increased, they noticed that Syntonics greatly expanded visual-field size, was very effective in treating functional vision problems, and frequently improved pathological conditions not directly treated.

In spite of increasing opposition from organized medicine, the College of Syntonic Optometry continued to grow. Then, the death of Dr. Spitler in 1961 threatened to bring the college to a sudden halt, as there was no one person who could immediately succeed him. However, a few of his followers, including Dr. J.O. Jenkins (one of Spitler's first students in 1933), Dr. Lowell Becraft, and Dr. Charles Butts, decided to keep the college and its teachings alive. These men were clinicians, not scientists, and they therefore began to unravel many of the mysteries about which Spitler had spoken and to develop highly practical clinical applications of them. Dr. Butts, responsible for rewriting Spitler's original work and creating the course that became the basis for today's Syntonics, became dean emeritus of the college. Dr. Jenkins, now at age 89, continues to manufacture instruments for syntonic application.

The 1970s brought a new generation of highly intuitive practitioners. These individuals, more correctly known as vision therapists rather than general optometrists, approached Syntonics very holistically, each bringing to it his or her own wisdom. Some were more interested in the research and technological aspects, while others focused on clinical applications. Dr. Robert Michael Kaplan, the first within this group to be published, reconfirmed that Syntonics could greatly enlarge the visual-field size of learning-disabled children.[9] Dr. John Downing, historically an inventor, developed new instrumentation. He combined traditional syntonic application with a new light source that flickered at different rates, thus entraining neurological rhythms during treatment.

As a member of this group, and having done a substantial amount of clinical work in this area, I soon noticed that Syntonics had a greater effect on people than had been spoken about by my colleagues or had been described in the literature. Although practitioners of this work had long been aware that learning ability improved following treatment, the specific areas of learning enhancement had not been identified, and the idea of treating eye diseases was almost never spoken about.

BREAKING THROUGH LEARNING BLOCKS:
THE EFFECTS OF SYNTONICS

In 1982 I began to take note of all the changes reported in my young patients by their parents and teachers, as well as the changes I perceived in my patients (from an optometric perspective) following their treatments. After several informal clinical investigations, I decided to conduct a controlled study on the isolated effects of syntonic (colored light) therapy on visual-field size, memory, and speed and accuracy of eye movements.[10] The research design called for a trained assistant to administer pre- and post-tests, as well as treatment. This reduced the possibility of my personal prejudice influencing the results. The study was limited to matched groups of referred subjects with academic difficulties, primarily in the area of reading. The experimental group looked at prescribed frequencies of light for 20-minute periods, four times per week for six weeks. The control group did not receive any colored-light treatment. None of the participants in either group were undergoing any other concurrent form of treatment such as prescriptive eyeglasses, vision therapy, tutoring, or psychological counseling. At the end of the six-week experimental period, both groups were retested with the following results:

1. The *visual field* increase for the experimental group was 208 times greater than for the control group;

2. The *visual attention span* increase for the experimental group was almost 4 times greater than for the control group;

3. The *visual memory* increase for the experimental group was 7 times greater than for the control group;

4. The *auditory memory* increase for the experimental group was 1.6 times greater than for the control group (although this was not statistically significant); and

5. The *eye movement* speed and accuracy did not change significantly.

Perhaps the most revealing information to come out of this study concerned areas that were not considered initially and that came particularly from the observations of parents and teachers. For example, those individuals whose visual fields were large to begin with showed greater improvement in all areas than did their counterparts whose visual fields were originally small. This finding is important in that it shows that Syntonics can effect statistically significant improvements in individuals with academic difficulties, regardless of their original visual-field size. In the daily logs kept by both parents and teachers of the children in the experimental group, the most common observations were that withdrawn children came out of their shells, hyperactive ones calmed down, and, in general, all the children became more open and receptive emotionally. Additionally, 75% of the subjects reported improvements in their school work, 40% showed visible improvement in their handwriting, and the only two participants who were on medication were able to totally eliminate their daily use of ritalin, a commonly used drug for calming hyperactive children.

SYNTONICS CASE STUDIES

After administering several thousand sessions and realizing the effectiveness of Syntonics in treating functional deficiencies in vision and learning, I decided to look at the possible application of Syntonics to disease. Having experienced its miraculous effects on my own mother's diseased eye condition early in my career, I now was ready to look further at the immense treatment possibilities available with this modality. Since treating eye diseases at that time was not commonly undertaken by optometrists, I decided to work with patients who were already medically diagnosed and had received whatever medical treatment was available. I made no claims for the treatment, worked along with the patient's physician whenever possible, and usually approached the work on a very short-term trial basis to assess its effectiveness. The more I worked, the more amazed I became with the results. Following are a few case histories to illustrate my experience. (Some of my patients' names have been changed to protect their privacy.)

Case 1

A few years ago, Robert, a close friend, came to my office seeking possible assistance with an eye disorder that he had been told might rob him of his vision. Then 37 years of age, Robert had been diagnosed as having had glaucoma for the previous five years. Glaucoma, an eye disease characterized by increased pressure in the eye, can, if not properly regulated by medication or surgery, lead to irreparable damage to the sensitive tissues of the eye, possibly resulting in blindness. Frequently, such excessively high pressures cause changes in the field of vision over time. In advanced cases, these changes are irreversible and greatly affect visual function. My friend Robert had an advanced case of this disease, and his left eye had lost a substantial portion of its field of vision, as seen in figure 27 (visual-field chart labeled "before").

I sent him home with a special mask housing a blue-green filter and instructed him to sit outside in the sunshine every day for 30 minutes wearing the mask. I had no idea if it would help, but since it was the same filter combination that so helped my mother, I decided to try it. I asked Robert to return in three weeks for an evaluation. To my surprise, when he returned his intraocular pressures had dropped and his visual field showed a definite improvement. Encouraged by these findings, we jointly decided to continue with the same treatment for a much longer period of time. After four months, Robert's intraocular pressures had dropped substantially. His visual field had expanded beyond my wildest hopes, and it had opened into areas that were thought to be impossible for someone with his condition. (See figure 27, visual-field chart labeled "after".)

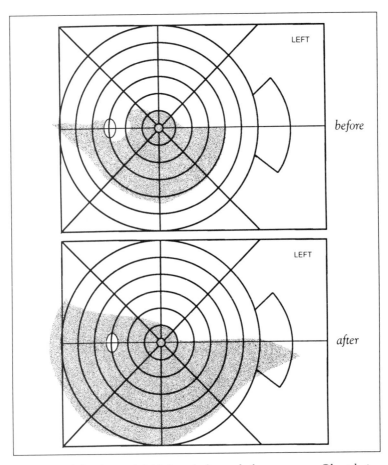

Figure 27. *Robert's visual-field charts before and after treatment. Chart design reprinted with permission from Dr. John Downing.*

Case 2

In 1986, a colleague called my office asking if I would do a visual evaluation on an elderly nonverbal, nonambulatory gentleman who had suffered a stroke. He told me that the family would gladly bring him to my office by ambulance. Understanding the fear someone in that condition would feel, I offered to conduct the evaluation in the man's home, thus allowing him the comfort and familiarity of his own "safe harbor."

Upon entering his home I was greeted by his wife, who introduced me to his nurse and took me to her husband's room. On the way to the room, the nurse told me that the physical therapist had totally given up on the man, as she had seen no improvement in him in more than six months. As I entered the room, the first thing that struck my eye was a metal "A"-frame-looking device similar to those used for removing engine blocks from cars. The device was obviously used for lifting the man into and out of bed.

When I was introduced to Anthony, he didn't so much as move his eyes in response. Eighty-four years old, clothed in a hospital gown and diaper, he looked like a man who had just been released from a long stay in a concentration camp. His body was rigid and convoluted, his eyes encrusted and half closed, and his body weight obviously lower than his age. Unsure as to how to begin, I placed my right hand on his chest, over his heart, and just stared into his eyes. Within a few seconds, his expression changed as if to say, "There is someone in here." On pure intuition, I decided to recommend two 20-minute sessions of Syntonics per day for the next three weeks, along with daily periods of sitting outside in the sunshine and fresh air. Based on an objective measurement, I also recommended a pair of glasses to be used for watching television. I brought over the equipment with appropriate instructions for the nurse and left for a two-week lecture circuit on the West Coast. Upon my return, there was a message from Anthony's wife stating that Anthony was trying to talk, was eating better, and was looking somewhat like his old self.

At the end of the three-week period, I went to evaluate the changes in Anthony, eager to satisfy my curiosity about his wife's message. When I arrived, I saw Anthony across the room in his wheelchair, reading his newspaper and turning the pages by himself. He apparently recognized me, for he said, "Nice to see you," grabbed my hand, shook it firmly, and smiled. I was blown away. His color was totally different, his eyes were clear, and obviously his brain was functioning. His wife told me that for the first time in eight months he was making sounds, occasionally speaking words, eating normally, moving more, requesting that his needs be met, and even showing her special affection. Upon further inquiry, she revealed most of his health history. In addition to Anthony's heart problems, diabetes, skin cancer, and previous periods of partial paralysis, he had suffered from at least fourteen strokes over the years. Anthony's wife was not fluent in English, so I asked his daughter to please write me a detailed letter describing any changes she had noticed due to the light treatment. Approximately three months later, I received a seven-page, typed letter from which the following is excerpted:

Dear Dr. Liberman:

At the beginning of February my brother suggested I contact you to see if you felt that Dad could use different glasses which would enable him to read and see TV with more ease. You were kind enough to come to my parent's place, check Dad's eyes, and recommend that he be given eyeglasses specifically for viewing the TV, and that he be put on a treatment involving light.

To be very frank with you, I was totally skeptical of what you were suggesting, but saw the benefit psychologically to both my parents. The first week of treatment reinforced my initial skepticism. There was very little noticeable change, and in addition, Mom had to hold Dad in position during the treatment (she put her head in the hood with him to make sure his eyes were open, and when they weren't she would pry them open and keep them that way).

Then, small things began to happen. Dad would stay awake longer; he would do his vocalization sounds more frequently (Mom was overjoyed that he was beginning to complain more). Dad's smile changed. It now said, "Hey, how are you—I'm sitting here not able to do anything, which I'm beginning to find amusing." His sense of humor was surfacing. He began to hear and react the first time we called his name. When he was in bed, he started to put his left arm on his head (very typical mannerism of Dad's), and he stayed awake longer. He was reacting more to his environment, particularly food. He would give definite indications of "nos" and "yeses" in terms of wanting more, or less, or liking or disliking something. When I would ask him a question, Dad now returned that look of understanding that was so intrinsically his. He would put his left arm on his forehead, lick his lips and say, "Well . . ." The entire response was so fluid and uniquely his, that I did double takes when nothing came after the "Well . . ."

By the time the third week of treatment rolled around, Mom kept saying "Antonio casi me hablo" (Anthony almost spoke to me). It became a daily thing. At one opportunity Mom, who had little time to think about her looks, was wearing a torn skirt. As she was moving Dad around, he pointed a finger (left arm) at the tear and raised his eyebrows as if to say, "Change that." He started doing this more frequently, initiating a conversation, but always the same way — pointing a finger and emitting a semi-grunt.

The biggest change I saw was in Paul, my husband. He had gone to my parents to build wheelchair ramps one evening. As he walked through the door, back from my parent's house, Paul looked at me in surprise and said, "I can't believe what has happened to your Dad." I was expecting the worst; I got a litany of Dad's vast improvement. Dad had recognized Paul as soon as he walked through the door, raised his left arm and shook Paul's hand. Paul, like I, saw such fluidity in action that he waited for Dad to respond to his hellos, which of course, did not come. Dad shook his hand firmly, not weakly. He was responding in a manner that Paul had thought Dad would never be able to do again.

Dad's appetite improved. The length of period he would stay awake increased. When he read the newspaper now, instead of waiting for me to turn the page or newspaper over, he would do it himself. Always very carefully, very deliberately. He would stay glued to the TV when a baseball game was being shown. He even tried to play with my three-year-old.

He was slowly, but surely, getting back some of what he had lost. I was hoping that as he remained more lucid, longer, he would then make a greater effort at relearning how to move his right side. Perhaps this would have been his next step in development, particularly since he was now handling bigger pieces of food without choking, which meant that if the swallowing mechanism was relearning, there was hope for another part of his body.

In looking back at the improvement in Dad after the light treatment (that is what we call it in the family), I can see where one thing seemed to have led to another. In other words, once a certain block was destroyed, or a door opened, the improvement never reached a stationary moment, but was building on itself and getting bigger and bigger. Being ignorant of medicine, and why the light treatment helped Dad, I can, however, positively say that it was the direct cause of the improvements he underwent toward the end of his life.

Case 3

This case involves a 47-year-old Austrian woman, who, while visiting the United States, called me regarding possible treatment for an eye condition that had been diagnosed when she was 20. Her condition, retinitis pigmentosa, is thought to be hereditary and is usually evident at an early age. It progressively affects certain photosensitive elements (the rods) of both eyes, producing defective night vision, visual-field loss, central vision loss (by middle age), and, frequently, total blindness. Currently, no effective treatment is known.

The patient told me that she first noticed difficulty with night driving at the age of 20, and that at the present time she could not walk alone at night. Sensing a possible long-term emotional component to her condition, I asked her about her childhood. She said that she was raised by her grandmother. As an only child, she had an unhappy childhood and rarely saw either of her parents at home.

A report from a previous (1984) ophthalmological evaluation revealed a very constricted visual field of only 8 degrees and indicated that she would be fortunate to retain useful vision beyond the age of 55 or 60. My evaluation revealed a 10-degree field, confirming the previous finding. Since she was staying approximately a hundred miles from my office and was planning to return to Austria in exactly two weeks, I recommended fourteen days of self-treatment at home. At the end of the two weeks, her visual field had expanded to 33 degrees in the right eye and 42 degrees in the left. She also mentioned that she was reading better, occasionally walking at night by herself, and in general feeling great. Her husband enthusiastically agreed.

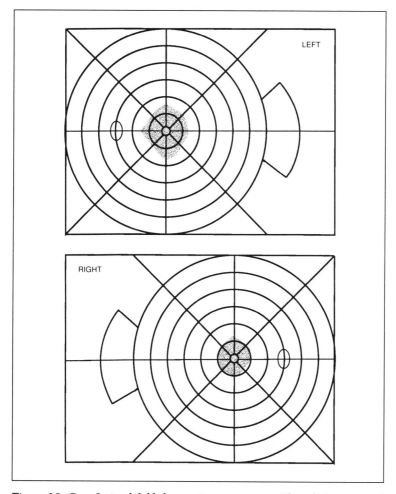

Figure 28. *Case 3 visual-field charts prior to treatment. Chart design reprinted with permission from Dr. John Downing.*

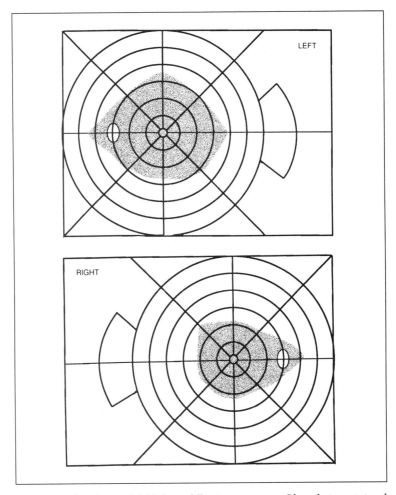

Figure 29. *Case 3 visual-field charts following treatment. Chart design reprinted with permission from Dr. John Downing.*

Summary

These cases are not presented to prove that light therapy would be effective in all cases of glaucoma, stroke, or retinitis pigmentosa, but so that all of us may realize that "the sky is the limit" until proven otherwise. It is important to realize that if we don't stretch our belief systems about what conditions are treatable and what forms of treatment are effective, many of us may prematurely greet the end of our lives as a result of having an attitude that "there's nothing that can be done for us."

If light therapy is effective in treating functional vision problems, learning deficits, and certain eye diseases, what other conditions might it help? Since most learning occurs visually, and since the eyes seem to be the major entryway for light into the body, what would be the effect of modifying general lighting and/or environmental color in the academic environment?

8

Light, Color & Learning

Previous chapters have mentioned the studies of several researchers whose findings clearly showed that cool-white fluorescent lighting, which is used in most classrooms, creates bodily stress and thus interferes with learning ability. These studies also showed that lighting more closely simulating sunlight (full-spectrum fluorescent lighting) creates little or no stress and improves behavior and academic achievement. Additionally, research by Gerard, Wohlfarth, and others indicated that certain colors have a measurable and predictable effect upon humans.

WOHLFARTH'S SCHOOL STUDIES

Based on these and other findings, Dr. Harry Wohlfarth decided to arrange a series of experiments to evaluate the effects of light and/or color on certain physiological, behavioral, and academic variables within a school setting.[1] In 1981, he and his associate Catherine Sam conducted a study at the Elves Memorial Child Development Centre, a school for handicapped children in Edmonton, Alberta, Canada. They evaluated the combined impact of selected colors and full-spectrum lighting on the behavior and physiology of both blind children with severe behavioral disorders and sighted children with severe handicaps. Physiology and behavior were monitored and measured before and after full-spectrum lighting was installed and classroom walls were painted with selected shades of warm colors. The decision to repaint the walls was based on the work of Ertel, who found that the use of bright warm colors such as yellow and orange improved the intelligence quotient (IQ) and academic achievement of school-age children.[2]

The results were *highly significant*. In the newly painted rooms with full-spectrum lighting, systolic blood pressure dropped an average of 20 points per child, and behavior (especially the reduction of aggression) improved dramatically. However, when the full-spectrum lighting was changed back to the original cool-white fluorescent tubes, blood pressure increased and the children once again became disorderly. Another very interesting finding was that the *blind subjects were as affected as the sighted ones.*

Although this study confirmed the psychophysiological and behavioral effects of light and color, the effects of color could not be distinguished from those of light. In order to make this distinction clear, Wohlfarth designed a new, comprehensive study in which he evaluated more variables simultaneously than had previously been attempted. During the 1982-1983 school year, he concurrently conducted several different research studies at four similarly matched elementary schools in Wetaskiwin, Alberta, Canada.[3-6] He substituted warm shades of light yellow and light blue wall paint for the original orange, white, beige, and brown wall paints, and replaced the cool-white fluorescent lights with full-spectrum ones. The purpose of the study was to evaluate the effects of different environmental light and/or color conditions on systolic blood pressure, mood states, absences due to illness, total disciplinary incidences, classroom noise levels, IQ test scores, and academic performance over a full year of school. Different variables were assigned to each school as follows:

1. School number 1 was selected as a control and was therefore left in its original condition;

2. School number 2 had both its lighting and wall colors changed;

3. School number 3 had only its lighting changed; and

4. School number 4 had only its wall colors changed.

The results were quite impressive. The best results for all areas evaluated, except discipline, were in school number 2, where both lighting and wall color were changed. The worst results were consistently found in school number 1, where neither lighting nor color were changed. In school number 2, students were less stressed, quieter, less moody, showed the greatest improvement on combined academic and IQ tests scores, and were absent due to illness only one-third as often as the children in school number 1. Total disciplinary incidences were lowest in school number 4, where only wall color was changed. Remember that these changes were charted over a complete school year, which significantly reduced the chances of error. With such impressive results, along with the fact that Dr. Wohlfarth is considered one of the world's leading color researchers, one wonders why all children's classrooms are not designed with such warm colors and full-spectrum lighting. (See appendix C: colors used in Wohlfarth's experiments.)

VITALE'S OBSERVATIONS

Although the general field of education has not yet "seen the light" that Wohlfarth and others kindled, many teachers have intuitively understood for a long time the powerful influence of light and color. Barbara Meister Vitale, a well-known educator, lecturer, and author of such works as *Unicorns Are Real: A Right-Brained Approach to Learning,* and *Free Flight: Celebrating Your Right Brain,* has used color in her work since 1970. Recalling her personal observations, as well as those of other teachers with whom she had worked, she wrote the following in a letter to me:

1. Placing appropriately colored pieces of felt within the visual work space of a child frequently reduces hyperactivity, increases attention span, and improves the speed and accuracy of completing assignments. In most cases, the color red seems to be the most effective for reducing activity levels.

2. Behavioral changes are sometimes noticed in children when they wear different colored clothing.

3. By writing with different colored markers or putting words on different colored paper, some children and adults experience an increase in reading fluency, fewer pronunciation errors, and improved comprehension. They also experience an increase in long-term recall when notes are taken in their favorite color.

4. Some adults and children respond very well to reading or working under a blue light.

5. Adults and children who have difficulty with letter and word reversals, frequent loss of place, and/or words appearing to float above the page, respond very well to having a specific colored transparency placed over their reading material. This alone can sometimes drastically change their reading levels.

6. Nonreaders, when asked to visualize their favorite color, can frequently begin reading at the level of instruction they have been exposed to.

7. The value of color seems to be individual specific. In most cases, the color that works most effectively is either the person's favorite color or the color that is opposite on the color wheel.

IRLEN'S TINTED LENSES

If light and color can significantly improve the learning and behavior of normal children and adults, what might be its effect on individuals with learning difficulties? The effects of color on learning ability received wide publicity as a result of the work of Helen Irlen, a California psychologist.[7-11] She made her world debut May 15, 1988, on television's "60 Minutes," which aired a feature segment called "Reading by the Colors." Millions of people watched as Irlen performed magic before their eyes by transforming nonreading learning-disabled individuals into fluid readers. Irlen described her newly discovered form of "visual dyslexia," Scotopic Sensitivity Syndrome, and explained that the condition is caused by light that, when received by the eyes, actually distorts what the eyes see. Individuals suffering from this condition respond inappropriately to specific wavelengths of light; they feel overwhelmed in the presence of those wavelengths, almost as if they are allergic to them. Irlen's technique basically involves using colored transparencies and lenses to modify the light entering the eyes, thus eliminating the distortions perceived. The technique utilizes a trial-and-error approach in which the client subjectively chooses the pair of tinted lenses that creates the greatest improvement. Although the exact mechanism of action is unknown, Irlen feels that the prescribed tinted lenses (of which there are approximately 140 possible choices) selectively reduce or eliminate those wavelengths that the eyes cannot handle and transmit those wavelengths that the eyes can handle.

The basis for Irlen's technique, however, is not new, even in its present form. For the past 58 years, the College of Syntonic Optometry has been using selected light frequencies to treat learning disabilities and other problems by way of the eyes. Furthermore, Dr. Richard Frenkel, a physician from Scarsdale, New York, has utilized tinted lenses to treat psychiatric disorders for many years, in a manner somewhat similar to the system used by Irlen to treat learning problems.

The jury is still out on the Irlen lenses — not so much on whether they create an effect or not, but on what they are really doing when they are prescribed in isolation. The system raises many questions: How long does a specific treatment remain effective if it is used on a daily basis? Does the body build up a tolerance to the tint? What really happens when the body is radically restricted to a specific light-diet and only a selected portion of the spectrum is allowed to enter the eyes? What are the long-term effects on the wearers? In a recent study reported by the *Journal of the Royal Society of Medicine*, it was found that medical patients who had no eye diseases but wore tinted spectacles were more likely to be psychopathic than those who did not wear tinted spectacles.

ARE WE TREATING A CAUSE OR AN EFFECT?

Any treatment should be considered from the perspective of whether it is aimed at the *cause* of the problem or the *effect* of the problem. Having been a nonreading, hyperactive child with all the symptoms of a learning disability, I can fully appreciate how miraculous it would have felt to me as a child if I had been, all of a sudden, able to read easily. The real question, however, is what caused me to shut down that part of my learning ability as a child. Why was it that most of the children with whom I went to school didn't like school? Could our teaching methods, or the high demands placed on children to learn to read early, have something to do with their learning problems? Having worked with thousands of children and adults with learning difficulties, it has become increasingly evident to me that *they all show signs of fear.* Is it the learning difficulty that causes the fear or the fear that causes the learning difficulty? And if the latter, what causes the fear?

For years we have been labeling and relabeling children who appear to have difficulties we do not understand. We test and tutor them continually, only to find out that they are usually very bright but that for some reason outside of our understanding they do not achieve in the expected manner within the traditional learning environment. Although the labels for these children have changed from dumb, stupid, and lazy to dyslexic, minimally brain dysfunctioned, and learning disabled, the labels nonetheless scar them for life. Einstein, Beethoven, and Edison were thought to be either hopeless, stupid, or mentally slow. How many more of these so-called learning-disabled individuals will it take to show us that what we think describes a learning problem may really be characteristic of a different creative expression of intelligence? Also, many truly brilliant individuals consistently achieve below their potential level because they get frightened and freeze up in an academic environment.

We are beginning to discover that there are many different forms of intelligence, perhaps the least common of which is the one to which our educational system primarily caters. When will we realize that what we think is the problem frequently has nothing to do with what the *real* problem is? Which is more devastating: the so-called learning problem or the extreme personal violation children must feel when they are labeled or continually checked to uncover what is wrong with them? Do most of these children, who frequently become successful adults, really have a learning problem? Or does our culture have a problem seeing what is really going on? I believe it is the latter.

Since we were infants, most of us were made to feel as though we were incomplete in some way. If we could only try harder, be more like our older brothers or sisters, pay more attention, speak less, concentrate more, behave better, make better grades, and so on, we might then be OK. With all this going on, how could we have believed that there was truly nothing wrong with us? A real paradox of the newly uncovered syndromes is that they only add to our already existing personal lists of what is wrong with us. The question now is how we can use color to heal us deeply rather than to be just a temporary compensatory tool. This question is at the heart of my own work and research, and it will be addressed in part 3.

Up to this point, I have discussed the effects of light and color primarily on such psychophysiological functions as behavior, mood, learning, and certain pathologies. What about their effect on life-threatening illnesses? Will they respond to something as subtle as light? Can light be the medicine of the future?

9

A New Light on Cancer

Research consistently has shown that artificial light that simulates sunlight supports the body's light-dependent functions. Compared to other artificial light, it lowers bodily stress, resulting in improved health, mood, behavior, and learning. Based on this information, we need to broaden our concepts regarding the purpose of light. Light can no longer be thought of as merely a technological advancement used to illuminate our environment, but *must be embraced as potentially one of the most powerful disease-prevention tools at our disposal.*

LIGHT AND LONGEVITY

The pioneering work of Dr. John Ott illustrates the ability of light to affect health.[1] In 1964, Ott conducted experiments showing that mice living under pink fluorescent light were more likely to develop cancer and reproductive problems. To confirm the accuracy of Ott's findings, researchers at the National Institute of Environmental Health Sciences undertook extensive research on a special strain of mice bred to develop tumors.[2] Divided into three groups, the mice were assigned to live in separate environments, each one lighted by a different kind of fluorescent light. One light was pink, as in Ott's experiments, the second was cool white, and the third was daylight-simulating full spectrum.

The group living under the pink fluorescents were the first to develop tumors (after 42 weeks), just as Ott reported. The cool-white and full-spectrum groups developed tumors in 47 and 51 weeks, respectively. After 573 days, each group of mice seemed to develop a different level of resistance to cancer. Considering that many cancers are fatal, the fact that there was quite a difference between the time it took for tumors to develop in the pink group (42 weeks) versus the full-spectrum group (51 weeks) can be interpreted as implying that there may some day be significantly longer life spans for humans suffering from cancer. Dr. Spitler also found that rabbits living under different colors of light developed a host of pathological conditions. It is evident that the lighted environment affects development, level of health, and longevity.

To further illustrate this point, consider the work of Dr. Joan Smith-Sonneborn, a professor of zoology and physiology at the University of Wyoming who has been doing some ground-breaking research on the prevention of cancer and age damage to cells.[3-5] Her work is based on previous research indicating that in order for a cell to become cancerous it must first sustain damage to its hereditary blueprint (DNA). She noticed that the incidence of cancer increases with age, suggesting that the older people are, the greater is the likelihood for them to have accumulated the DNA damage that precedes cancer. Using single-celled organisms called paramecia, she was able to demonstrate that old cells do actually show an accumulation of DNA damage.

Her next inquiry was as to whether this damage could be repaired or possibly prevented. After speaking with Dr. Ron Hart, who had demonstrated that cancer caused in fish by certain types of ultraviolet (UV) radiation could be prevented if the UV damage was repaired, Dr. Smith-Sonneborn proceeded to investigate this idea further. Having already exposed her paramecia to far-ultraviolet radiation (UV-C, a bacteriocidal light), which caused DNA damage and also shortened the cells' life spans, she wished to see whether repairing this damage would actually reverse the accelerated aging caused by the exposure. She therefore exposed the damaged cells to near-ultraviolet radiation (UV-A) and found that the cells not only repaired themselves but also reversed their aging.

This in itself was dramatic, but what followed was no less than *miraculous*. After repairing these previously damaged cells with UV-A radiation, Dr. Smith-Sonneborn then wanted to see what would happen if she exposed them *once again* to the UV-A radiation. What she found was that the second exposure extended the life span of the cells by up to 50%, compared with the cells in the control group. Her findings clearly showed that certain types of light are not only capable of assisting cells in repairing their DNA, but also have the ability to stimulate life-extending capabilities within the DNA.

What does Dr. Smith-Sonneborn's discovery mean to the science of human disease prevention and longevity, especially if it is discovered that human cells have the same capabilities? Obviously, light is important to optimum health and disease prevention. It also can be used in the treatment of life-threatening diseases.

A DEATH RAY FOR CANCER: PHOTODYNAMIC THERAPY

In the year 1900, scientists first noticed that certain substances such as eosin, the pigment in red ink, were damaging to living tissue when exposed to visible light but were not toxic in the dark.[6] They found that some microorganisms, for instance, would be killed if they were exposed to specific dyes and then to light. At about this time, the French briefly made use of this early discovery to treat skin tumors in humans.[7]

It was later discovered that many of the compounds with this characteristic came from a family of light-activated chemicals called *porphyrins*. Although porphyrins are essential to almost all life forms on Earth and are intricately involved in such important processes as the formation of chlorophyll and hemoglobin, these life-giving chemicals, in excess, can become life threatening.[8] An example of this is a congenital disease called *porphyria*, which is caused by an excessive build-up of porphyrins in the body. People with this condition can experience severe pathological reactions and substantial damage to body tissues merely by exposing themselves to sunlight. The effects of light exposure are so physically destructive and visually grotesque that individuals with this condition can only venture out during the night. Incidentally, it is thought that this condition causes a bodily appearance that resembles the medieval descriptions of werewolves.[9]

In 1942, researchers noticed that, under certain conditions, tumors would fluoresce under light after porphyrins had been administered into the body. This discovery took on a new meaning for medicine when scientists at the Mayo Clinic found that porphyrins also accumulated in cancer cells.[10] In other words, cancer cells not only selectively take up porphyrins, but also fluoresce a brilliant red when activated by ultraviolet light, thus letting us know where they are hiding.

Combining these discoveries, researchers have come up with one of the most promising developments in cancer research in the last 20 years. It is a new technique, known as photodynamic therapy (PDT), which is the direct result of pioneering research over the last two decades by Dr. Thomas Dougherty at Roswell Park Memorial Institute in Buffalo, New York.[11-15] Photodynamic therapy became possible when it was discovered that certain intravenously injected photosensitive chemicals not only accumulate in cancer cells but selectively identify these cells under ultraviolet light and then exclusively destroy them when activated by red light. In other words, this technique can be used for both diagnosis and treatment. If the cells that have taken up the photosensitive chemicals give off a characteristic red glow under ultraviolet light, they are designated as cancerous.[16] No glow means there is no cancer. Red light is specifically used because of its longer wavelength, which allows it to penetrate tissue more deeply than blue light, which has a shorter wavelength.

Using a photosensitive chemical called Hpd and red light from an ordinary slide projector, Dougherty successfully eradicated his first tumor in a patient in 1973. Although Hpd was used in most of Dougherty's original research, today's most common, and only FDA-approved, photosensitive chemical for human use is called DHE, or Photofrin.[17] A purified form of Hpd, Photofrin is used not only to destroy targeted cancer cells but at times to actually locate cancerous tissue prior to destroying it. During the procedure, the patient is injected intravenously with a calculated amount of Photofrin, which is then allowed to circulate in the body while the patient is protected from direct sunlight or other bright lights. Although Photofrin was originally thought to accumulate only in cancerous tissue, it is now known that it also collects in certain normal tissues, including the kidneys, liver, spleen, and pancreas. For this reason, there is a 24- to 72-hour waiting period prior to treatment with light, in order to permit time for some of the Photofrin to clear out of normal tissues.[18]

The actual light used for this process is a specifically tuned red light of 630 nanometers.[19] (Remember that a nanometer is a unit of measurement for the wavelength of electromagnetic radiation and is equivalent to one billionth of a meter.) This red light is delivered from an argon-pumped laser directly to the treatment site via hair-thin fiberoptic tubes. Fiberoptic technology is specifically used because of its efficient light-conducting capabilities. In addition, the ease of insertion of the fiberoptic tubes into small bodily openings such as the urethra (the tiny tube through which the bladder empties) makes it possible to reach deeper and more difficult areas.

Within hours of the light treatment, the cancer cells begin to die, leaving most normal tissues unharmed. Even in tissues that are just partially cancerous, only the cancerous portions of the tissue will die. Since specific photosensitive dyes are combined with highly tuned laser light, the treatment is extremely precise. These photosensitive dyes could be likened to very sensitive planted grenades with light-triggered fuses.[20] Or, the cancer cells could be compared to a red balloon, which is inside a white balloon representing normal tissue; inside the red balloon is another white balloon, also representing normal tissue. The red laser light, focused on the middle red balloon, can burst this red balloon (the cancerous tissue) while leaving the inner and outer white balloons (normal tissue) intact.

To date, more than 3,000 people worldwide, with a wide variety of malignant tumors, have been experimentally treated with this technique with a high degree of efficacy and relative safety. Although they had been treated previously with surgery, chemotherapy, radiation, immunotherapy, or a combination of these, their tumors responded positively to the light treatment 70% to 80% of the time, *after only one treatment*.[21]

Photodynamic therapy is relatively simple, is painless, and has a higher degree of success in treating localized cancers than conventional treatments. However, its major limitation is that certain tumors, because of their depth or size, cannot be reached by the light. As long as the tumor can be reached, the treatment is almost always effective.[22] There is only one unpleasant side effect: Since light-activated Photofrin temporarily collects in the skin, patients frequently experience a high degree of sensitivity to sunlight and may possibly be susceptible to serious skin irritation for the first four to six weeks following treatment. These minor limitations, however, are presently being addressed and will most likely be resolved within the next few years. New photosensitive chemicals are presently being investigated that do not cause extended photosensitivity problems and will absorb longer wavelengths of light, thus penetrating tissue better.[23]

Photodynamic therapy has taken awhile to develop credibility. However, throughout the world it is now demanding the attention of physicians and medical researchers involved in the treatment of disease. Currently this technique is being evaluated in approximately 70 different centers worldwide, 45 of them in the United States and Canada.[24] (See appendix D for a partial directory.) According to Dr. Dougherty, a pioneer in this technology, photodynamic therapy will probably receive approval for general use in Canada during 1990 and in the United States by the end of 1991. While the effectiveness of this technique is now being compared against conventional treatments in cancers of the esophagus, lung, and bladder, it is also being used to treat gynecological, colo-rectal, and metastatic breast cancers, as well as those affecting the skin, brain, eye, head, and neck. It shows great promise as a tool for the early detection and simple nonintrusive treatment of cancers that might not otherwise be detected.[25]

The treatment of a number of other health conditions with photodynamic therapy is currently being investigated. Venereal warts, which

have now become epidemic, probably will be treated by the topical application of Photofrin followed by nonlaser red-light treatment. It is
presently thought that this treatment may actually rid the body of the
venereal wart virus if it is not systemic. Another very promising area
of future research is the use of photodynamic therapy in the treatment
of atherosclerotic plaques. These plaques, the result of a gradual build-
up of fatty deposits (mainly cholesterol) on the inner lining of the
arterial walls, cause a progressive narrowing of these vessels, thus decreasing blood flow to vital organs. If these deposits get too large, they
can totally obstruct the flow of blood through arteries, possibly leading
to heart attacks, strokes, or even death. Recent animal studies have
shown that Photofrin collects in atherosclerotic plaques and that,
when it is activated with low levels of light, it literally *melts* these
plaques away. If similar results can be reproduced in humans, this treatment may significantly reduce the incidence of heart attacks and
strokes, and may even eliminate the need for coronary bypass surgery
in some cases.

LIGHT: THE BLOOD CLEANSER

Aside from the present use of light in the treatment of cancer, its
potential applications for blood banking and AIDS research are very
promising.[26] During the last few years, scientists at Baylor University
Medical Center have used light to destroy viruses causing AIDS and
other infectious diseases. Under the leadership of Dr. Lester Matthews,
director of the Baylor Research Foundation, new technology is being
developed that could decontaminate blood for transfusions, eliminating the risk of transfusion infections from viruses such as those that
cause herpes and AIDS.[27] Using the same photosensitive chemical
(Photofrin) and red light used by Thomas Dougherty, Lester Matthews
and other researchers have been able to kill 100% of viruses causing
herpes simplex type 1 (cold sores), measles, AIDS, and other illnesses,
without any evidence of damage to normal blood elements.[28] These
researchers believe that photodynamic therapy can be effective against
all viruses encased in viral envelopes, including those causing hepatitis,

AIDS, and some forms of leukemia.[29] The most encouraging aspect of this technology is that it can selectively destroy viruses and other impurities without harming the blood itself. This is a major advancement in blood-decontamination technology. Present blood-screening techniques are less than 100% effective, since in rare cases certain viruses are not detectible even though they are present.

TUNABLE LASERS

Although Matthews's original work, including killing the AIDS virus, was accomplished with a regular, nonlaser light source, future research will probably make use of special tunable lasers now being used by scientists working in the United States government's Strategic Defense Initiative (SDI) program.[30,31] I can foresee that, in the near future, photodynamic therapy, alone or in combination with other conventional techniques, will be able to successfully treat most, if not all, cancers and other life-threatening diseases. The technique will probably become as common as microsurgery for knee injuries.

Imagine a patient with a hard-to-reach large tumor. After intravenous injection with the appropriate photosensitizer, a small incision is made near the tumor site and two fiberoptic probes are simultaneously inserted. One probe is connected to a video camera that allows the surgeon immediate visual access to the suspected site, while the other is connected to a tunable laser that sends the desired wavelength of light directly to the targeted point. Once the site of the tumor has been determined by the fluorescing of the tissue, the appropriate wavelength of light can be used to treat the affected area and thus destroy the cancer.

A further step would be completely noninvasive treatment. This might involve a device that could accurately measure the precise location of the tumor and the distance from the skin to its site in the body. It might also involve a laser that not only could be tuned to the appropriate wavelength but also to the exact depth of penetration. Does this sound a bit like the activities of Dr. McCoy on "Star Trek"? I am sure that this technology exists in our not-too-distant future.

Another possible scenario is an annual light bath along with a person's yearly physical examination. Imagine receiving an injection of a photosensitive chemical that accumulates *only* in cancer cells and does not create any problems with photosensitivity. Diagnosis would not be necessary, as merely receiving the therapeutic light bath would rid the body of any cancerous tissue, regardless of its stage of development. Possibly, the injection wouldn't even be needed, and light itself would provide the rebalancing necessary to restore health. The light treatment could also address both the physical and emotional components of disease simultaneously. I will discuss these possibilities in part 3.

10

Light: Nature's Miracle Medicine

From the time of early historical accounts to the present day, people have recognized that cyclic or rhythmic patterns are an integral part of the functioning of all dynamic systems. Originating at a level probably outside of our own universe, these cycles affect all other dynamic systems residing within our universe. In a stair-step or dominolike manner, the cosmic cycles affect our universe, which then affects the solar system, which then affects the Earth, and so on down through Earth's climate, seasons, inhabitants, right down to the smallest particle within an atom. Since all things are integrally connected in this way, everything affects everything else. Nothing escapes this process.

The purpose of these introductory comments is to develop a foundation upon which to build a better understanding of how the cycles of our human lives relate to the cycles of our environment. What, for example, do the seasons describe? How does the activity of each season affect our lives during that season? If we are truly meant to be one with the universe, shouldn't our lifestyles be synchronized with nature? What would that experience really be like? How does our lack of synchronicity with the universe affect us?

Since the time of Hippocrates, it has been known that human beings, like animals, have specific daily and seasonal rhythms. As a matter of fact, Hippocrates himself thought this to be so important that he recommended that all individuals who wished to study medicine should first become fully aware of seasonal changes and the coin-

cidental changes within animals and humans.[1] By understanding
seasonal variations, students can better understand the physiological
and emotional changes associated with them. For instance, certain
psychological and physical disorders seem to be more prevalent in the
fall, while human fertility seems to reach a peak during the summer.

I believe that these universally occurring variations affect all living things. Plants and animals awaken in the spring of the year, develop
and mature in the summer, slow down in the fall, and rest in the
winter. I believe that people are meant to respond to the seasons in
an identical manner. Consider our responses to the seasons: we want
to begin anew by doing spring cleaning; we experience a childlike
summer-camp mentality when we take time away from our usual rou-
tines to have the opportunity to grow and expand unobstructively; we
take slow walks as we experience the beauty of fall; we feel coldness
and stillness during the very dead of winter.

There is great importance in the messages conveyed to us by the
seasons. Spring has always been a time to revive and summer a time
to fulfill. Fall clearly describes maturity verging on decline, while
winter is nature's way of clearing off the old and creating a foundation
for a fresh start. Spring and summer define and create externalization,
a time for growth, movement, and fruition, whereas fall and winter
encourage internalization, a gradual slowing down, a time for quiet
introspection and rest.

Winter is specifically a time of year when we go within our homes
as well as our psyches — natural settings for deep feelings to arise and
families to reconnect, followed by maturation of expression and resolu-
tion. It is truly nature's time to look deeply inside and *heal the heart*.
It is as if nature has a master plan for us to spend part of our lives exploring our external environments, and part of our lives exploring our
internal environments. Unfortunately, winter, which was once a time
of year when nature assisted our inner growth by supporting us in
going into the unlit aspects of our souls, has now become a time of
depression and sadness dreaded by many.

A CONDITION KNOWN AS SAD

A general slowing down and lowering of mood and enthusiasm in association with winter has been noticed globally for thousands of years. Although most people feel some degree of internal change in response to the cold, shortened days of winter, many people experience changes that trigger serious debilitating depression and in some cases may cause them to become suicidal. In the last ten years, scientists at the National Institute of Mental Health have described an emotional disorder characterized by drastic mood swings and depression that arrive in the winter and leave in the spring.[2] Unlike most individuals suffering from depression, people with this disorder (four times as many women as men) do not lose sleep or their appetite. Instead, they eat more (especially carbohydrates), sleep more, are less interested in sex, gain weight, frequently become withdrawn, and in general undergo a change in personality.[3] It's as though they are in a state of seasonal hibernation, or temporarily living in a cocoon. Some sufferers have even stated that they feel as if they should have been bears.

Although it has been scientifically understood for only a short period of time, it is estimated that nearly 25 million people in the United States alone feel the effects of this disorder, now called "Seasonal Affective Disorder," or SAD.[4] How is it possible that so many people are presently afflicted with a condition that has just in the last ten years come into medical awareness? Dr. Norman E. Rosenthal, who first identified the symptoms in 1981 and named this disorder SAD, feels that because the condition is so common, its symptoms are accepted as normal.

TREATING SADness WITH LIGHT

It has now been discovered that people with this disorder are actually suffering from *sunlight starvation* and can be assisted greatly by merely letting a little light into their lives. J.F. Cauvin, in 1815, wrote,

> The influence of light on the morale of man is very powerful. The physician will prescribe sun for the sad and the weak. When taken

with moderate exercise, it will revive lost courage. The rich people of England and Germany go to the south of France and Italy to cure the disease of temper called spleen; or at least to get away from the monotony of an almost continuing climate.[5]

To help explain some of the physiological mechanisms underlying this condition and its treatment, I will reiterate the functions of the pineal gland. Located deep in the brain's core, the pineal is a very important organ that plays a highly significant role in the regulation of the body's vital functions. Although much of the scientific literature states that the pineal has different functions in humans than in other species, I believe that its functions are identical in most species. If there *is* a difference in the function of the pineal between humans and other species, it is probably created by the amount of artificial lighting used in our society as well as by how out of touch most people are with their environment. In addition to the fact that the pineal regulates the onset of puberty, induces sleep, and influences our moods, it acts as the body's light meter and timer, orchestrating our internal functions and synchronizing them with the external environment of nature. Since the pineal is primarily regulated by environmental light changes, we are artificially manipulating and desensitizing its function much of the time by the widespread use of artificial lighting in our indoor and outdoor environments.

Another very important aspect of pineal function is that its effects on our physiology and mood are mediated by the daily rhythmic secretion of its hormone, melatonin, which is highest at night and lowest during the day. The significance of melatonin's regular daily rhythm was not fully recognized until 1980, when Dr. Alfred Lewy and Dr. Thomas Wehr discovered that bright light could suppress the normal nighttime secretion of melatonin.[6] Their discovery not only explained melatonin's cyclic nature, but also proved that the light of day suppresses melatonin's secretion while the darkness of night increases it. Based on this discovery as well as the observations of other clinical researchers and the positive results found in some initial pilot studies, a basic hypothesis was formulated. Lewy and Wehr suggested that lengthening a winter day with bright artificial light *could trick the brain into thinking it was spring*, and thus alleviate the depression created by the short days of winter. This hypothesis was based on the knowledge that the secretion of melatonin regulates seasonal rhythms in animals and that the hypothalamus (one of the places where light information goes from the eyes) is responsible for controlling many of the functions that are disturbed in depressed individuals.

In their need to validate the existence of this form of depression as well as the effectiveness of their proposed treatment, Drs. Wehr and Rosenthal began searching for individuals who had specific seasonal symptoms. After reviewing thousands of cases, they realized that virtually all these people were describing the same symptoms as the individuals in their initial pilot studies. The time had arrived for a more comprehensive study.

An initial controlled study was designed for two groups of seasonally depressed patients.[7] Each group was treated for two weeks, six hours a day, with either bright full-spectrum light or dim yellow light. Each group was then exposed for another two-week period to the light source with which they had not yet been treated. This study was designed as a double blind so that none of the scientists, aside from the primary researcher, had any knowledge of the order of light treatment received by the patients. In addition, the patients were not aware of which light source was thought to be therapeutic.

The results were dramatic. All patients experienced significant improvements under the bright full-spectrum light treatment, while none showed improvements under the dim yellow light, even though that color is associated with the sun. Some patients under the full-spectrum bright light described themselves as being taken out of hibernation; others reported feeling wonderful, productive, and able to resume their normal activities.

The results of this initial study not only established the existence of Seasonal Affective Disorder and its effective treatment, but created a whole new approach to treatment that has now expanded well beyond the field of psychiatry. To date, the antidepressant effects of bright-light treatment have been scientifically documented by so many different controlled studies internationally that it is considered the treatment of choice for Seasonal Affective Disorder (SAD). (See appendix E: partial directory of practitioners and referral centers.) Based on all the existing research, some general statements can be made regarding Seasonal Affective Disorder and bright light treatment:

- SAD is an emotional disorder characterized by drastic mood swings, lowered energy, and depression that occur about the same time each year, arriving in the winter and vanishing in the spring. The further north people live, the more likely they are to experience winter depression. For example, while SAD affects only 8.9% of the residents of Sarasota, Florida, more than 30% of those living in Nashua, New Hampshire, are affected.[8] Although this condition is seen primarily in adults between the ages of 20 and 40, children have also been found to suffer from this affliction.[9] For them, the irritability, fatigue, and sadness are frequently accompanied by a decline in concentration and school performance.

- This condition, found more often in women than in men (four to one), is usually accompanied by overeating, excessive sleeping, weight gain, reduced sex drive, and sometimes a lowering of immune function.

- SAD is thought to arise in part from high levels of melatonin brought on by the shortened day length and less available daylight associated with winter.

- Although the exact mechanism of action is unknown, bright-light treatment by way of the eyes has been found to have significant antidepressant effects on more than 80% of those suffering from SAD or its milder form, called "winter blues."

- The amount of bright light used in treatment is very important, as certain levels of illumination have documented physiological effects:
  a) Exposure to bright light can rapidly reduce the levels of melatonin in the blood, which may be abnormally high at certain times of the day;

b) The time of day that treatment is given can advance or retard the body's biological clock, thereby affecting daily rhythms such as sleep patterns, body temperature, hormone secretion, and so on.

These shifts in the timing of the body's physiological functions may be the basis for light's therapeutic effect on this condition.

- The most widely accepted light source for the treatment of SAD utilizes six 40-watt full-spectrum fluorescent tubes that create the equivalent brightness of approximately 2,500 candles (approximately one-fortieth the brightness of a sunny summer day). Technically, this amount of brightness is referred to as 2,500 lux, with one lux equaling roughly one candle. New phototherapy units are now available that produce the equivalent of 10,000 lux, thus reducing the treatment time to as little as one half hour per day.[10] In the near future, portable units will be available that will be worn on the head like a visor, giving the patient the opportunity to be mobile while receiving the treatment. The most recent development being evaluated in SAD treatment is a computerized device that simulates the gradual onset and fading of dawn and dusk.[11] Developed by Dr. Michael Terman and coworkers, this new device works while the patient is in bed and thus takes less time out of his or her busy schedule. To date it provides the closest imitation of the light changes in nature.

- Although the optimal timing and duration of treatment varies among patients, morning exposure seems generally to be superior to evening exposure, and any amount of time from one-half hour to four hours of bright-light treatment per day may be effective, depending on the individual, where he or she lives, the climate, and the time of year. In order for treatment to be effective, it must be applied daily for the duration of time that environmental light levels are insufficient for that person.[12]

- Some people feel the positive effects of this treatment after the initial session. For most people it takes from two to four days for the effects to be noticeable. On the other hand, skipping the treatment for approximately two days will cause most symptoms to recur.

- Treatment is generally well accepted by patients, although temporary side effects such as eyestrain, headaches, edginess, and difficulty in sleeping are sometimes encountered. To date, no longterm side effects have been documented.

Some psychiatrists are also reporting good results in treating what they call "seasonal energy syndrome" (winter depression and summer agitation) with colored glasses.[13] They've found that while red glasses seem to work well with fall/winter depression, polarized blue-green glasses are recommended for spring/summer agitation.

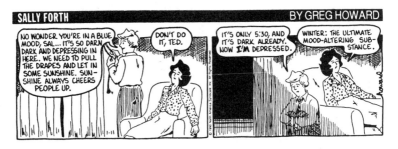

Figure 30. *Cartoon © by Greg Howard. Reprinted with special permission from North America Syndicate, Inc.*

Aside from the excellent clinical results being achieved with bright light in the treatment of SAD, several other areas of bright-light application are also being investigated. In a recent controlled study on nonseasonal depression, a group of California researchers, led by Dr. Daniel Kripke, found that bright-light treatment for three hours in the evening resulted in a small but statistically significant reduction in depression.[14] Bright-light therapy is also being evaluated as a possible treatment modality for certain patients with eating disorders such as bulimia, whose symptoms seem to worsen seasonally.[15] New evidence indicates that alcohol and drug detoxification may also be facilitated with bright light. A team of neurologists and psychiatrists in Austria tested 20 alcoholics with severe withdrawal symptoms. They found that those exposed to bright-light treatment for two days showed improvement in mood, ability to concentrate, and memory, and needed only 10% to 20% of the antianxiety medication required by those in the untreated group. Although research is sparse in this area, it appears that withdrawal symptoms may be alleviated in certain cases.[16]

Although the use of bright light in the treatment of certain aspects of alcoholism is relatively new, the relationship of light to this condition is not. In the July 30, 1971, issue of *Science* magazine, Dr. Irving Geller reported some highly significant findings that were the results of a somewhat accidental experiment.[17] While attempting to evaluate the effects of various types of stress on the development of alcoholism in rats, Dr. Geller noticed that the rats clearly preferred plain water during the week, but for unknown reasons went on alcoholic binges over the weekends. After some investigation, he discovered that the automatic timer switch regulating the on-off timing of the laboratory lights was malfunctioning. As a result, the rats were being left in continuous darkness over the weekends.

To determine whether it was the various stressors or the darkness that was causing the rats to prefer alcohol, Dr. Geller conducted another experiment. The results were very significant. He found that rats kept in total darkness and not subjected to any other stress preferred, over time, drinking water with alcohol in it to plain water. In order to further confirm his findings, Dr. Geller conducted one more experiment.

Recognizing that the pineal gland produces melatonin during darkness, Dr. Geller decided to evaluate the effects of melatonin injections on rats kept on a regular light-dark cycle and not subjected to any stress. This time he found that, even though the rats were kept on a regular light-dark cycle, the melatonin injections alone caused the rats to prefer water mixed with alcohol to plain water.

The results of Dr. Geller's experiments clearly show a significant relationship between reduced light levels and the development of alcoholism. The same relationship may be true for other types of chemical dependency.

HEALING SEXUAL DYSFUNCTIONS WITH LIGHT

Another medical application currently under investigation is the use of phototherapy in the treatment of sexual dysfunctions. It is widely accepted that all animals living in their natural environments breed on a seasonal basis and that the amount of light they see determines their reproductive status. As a matter of fact, each species has a specific requirement for the amount of light it must see in order to remain sexually competent. Since the pineal gland (the body's light meter) secretes melatonin as a way of cueing the organism about environmental light levels, it is obvious that melatonin has a profound effect on the reproductive physiology of any number of different animal species and most likely on that of humans as well.

It is now recognized that human sexual physiology is influenced by the pineal gland. High levels of melatonin (usually associated with short days) result in depressed sexual physiology (decreased sex hormone levels, slow sexual maturation), while low levels of melatonin (usually associated with long days) have the opposite effect.[18] This might be one reason why some children are experiencing early puberty in those highly developed countries (North America, Western Europe, and Japan) that use a tremendous amount of bright, artificial light.

In women with normal menstrual cycles, nighttime levels of melatonin are the lowest during ovulation and reach a peak during menstruation.[19] Women who never experience menses because of a condition known as hypothalamic amenorrhea exhibit abnormally high levels of melatonin for prolonged periods of time.[20] Melatonin not only suppresses ovulation in females but also sperm formation in males.[21] Since light suppresses melatonin synthesis, phototherapy may be a very simple, nonintrusive way to adjust abnormal situations affecting sexual physiology in both men and women. I can personally attest to its value in this area, as many of the women whom I treated for visual problems while I was in optometric practice coincidently experienced normalization of their menstrual cycles or reexperienced normal menstruation after many months of its absence.

Another very interesting discovery regarding melatonin is that it suppresses the growth of specific types of tumors in both humans and animals.[22] In women with certain types of breast tumors, nighttime levels of melatonin are very low. Also, animals that were administered daily melatonin developed such tumors much less often. If the growth of certain tumors can be suppressed by melatonin, which is directly affected by light, then we should be able to affect tumor development with light. Although the role that light plays in reproductive physiology and tumor development is only beginning to be understood, its future applications are vast.

RESETTING THE BODY'S INTERNAL CLOCK

Shift workers, problem sleepers, and even jet-lag sufferers may be in for a bright surprise in the near future. New research is indicating that the body's biological clock, which tells us when to sleep and when to be wide awake, is extremely sensitive to bright light and darkness.[23] Clinically, this means that subjecting people to precisely timed light exposures, by way of their eyes, may be helpful in resetting their bodies' primary internal timers, thus correcting sleep disorders, assisting shift workers in adjusting to new schedules, and helping travelers by reducing the symptoms associated with jet lag.[24] Another application of light now being evaluated is the correction of sleep disorders frequently found in patients with Alzheimer's disease.[25] These elderly individuals, averaging only half the daily exposure to bright sunlight as their healthy counterparts, are thought to be suffering from a disruption in their sleep/wake cycle due to a reduced exposure to light. Light therapy is presently being considered as a viable treatment. If these patients are able to sleep better at night, perhaps their cognitive ability would improve during the day. As stated in an old Italian saying, "Where the sun does not go, the doctor goes."

Imagine this new technology in our modern jetliners and airports! Perhaps during certain flights you will be instructed to pull down your window shade for a specific period of time while the entire aircraft is brightly illuminated, or while certain lights are turned on near your seat. This could significantly reduce your jet lag. Or, airports may have large rooms set up to treat you before or after your trip so that jet lag becomes a thing of the past. Although this technology is a few years away, researchers have some suggestions for today's long-distance travelers that, when followed, can adjust their internal clocks by up to three hours per day using everyday light and darkness:[26]

- Whether traveling east or west, avoid exposure to morning light (until about 10:00 a.m.) just prior to departure, during the flight, and after arrival. Although welder's goggles are recommended, very dark sunglasses should suffice for this purpose. Keep your glasses on and window shades drawn until at least 10:00 a.m. to avoid any sudden bursts of daylight.

- During those same days, maximize your exposure to afternoon and early-evening light. A window seat is recommended in order to assist in bright-light exposure during the flight.

- During afternoon flights, do not draw the cabin shades or watch an afternoon movie.

LIGHT AND DENTISTRY

One of the newest, state-of-the-art techniques in restorative dentistry involves the use of light-cured composite materials that closely resemble the natural color of teeth.[27] The use of silver fillings (considered toxic by many) seems to be declining as this new technology continues to improve.

Today's visit to the dentist is much easier and faster than it used to be. In the case of typical fillings, once the decay has been removed, the composite filling material is injected into the area being repaired by means of a hand-held "caulking gun" type of device. The dentist or assistant then shines a beam of visible light on the affected area, which cures the photo-activated composite material and results in a very functional and aesthetically pleasing restoration.[28]

NEEDLES OF LIGHT

Another futuristic approach to healing with light can be found in the field of acupuncture. This science, which for thousands of years primarily used only needles to stimulate acupuncture points, has in recent years utilized pulsing electrical currents, ultrasonic stimulation, high-frequency sound, and most recently laser light to accomplish similar results.[29] Even though needles are still used by most acupuncturists, *laserpuncture* is gaining great popularity. Developed by the Soviets, this technique involves the stimulation of acupuncture points by low-energy laser beams. Although this technology is still in its early stages, initial clinical results are suggesting that laserpuncture may be even more effective than the classical needling approach.

COLOR: THE BODY'S LIFE FORCE

Having studied the work of many noteworthy individuals whose research substantiates the value of light and color to our health, I am most impressed by those research clinicians whose own lives are living testimonials of their work. One such person, Dr. Hazel Parcells, holds doctorates in philosophy, chiropractic, and naturopathy; she is more than 100 years old, in excellent health, and continues to maintain an active private practice in Albuquerque, New Mexico.

For almost 40 years, Dr. Parcells has applied color in her holistic practice with consistently good results.[30] In patients who have suffered strokes, she finds that color can in many cases successfully eliminate paralysis and fully restore normal function. During the birth process, she applies color treatments to both mother and infant in order to reduce shock, hemorrhage, and recovery time. Additionally, she reports that these children have fewer health problems than those not receiving this treatment during delivery.

Dr. Parcells feels that color is the body's "life force." In cases of illness or exhaustion, she finds that the flow of color to the body's organs is reduced until health is restored. Color, she says, can change *any* function of the body.

NEUTRALIZING STRESS WITH COLOR

A very innovative psychotherapeutic application of light has been developed by Dr. Richard Frenkel, a psychiatrist from Scarsdale,

New York.[31-33] He has been investigating and clinically using color to treat human stress since the early sixties. After 25 years of clinical experience, Frenkel hypothesizes that stress is encoded in the mind as color. Since everything in life is colored, he feels that all of our experiences, as well as our reactions to them, are fused into what he calls an Experience Complex and then coded in the mind as specific colors. To Frenkel, the mind acts as a *computerized color information bank* that stores experiences, both stressful and nonstressful, in their respective colors.

Using a technique he calls "color refraction," Frenkel determines how a certain patient responds to different colors (red, orange, yellow, green, blue, purple, white, brown, and gray). He is primarily interested in which colors trigger old painful memories, resulting in stress. Once he determines which colors provoke these stressful responses, he then neutralizes the effects of the stress by having the patients look at them through appropriately tinted glasses. By wearing these glasses on a daily basis, the effects of these stress-producing colors are optically negated, thus reducing or eliminating the anxieties felt by the patients. He also uses a patented instrument called an "imagescope" and a technique that he calls "image analysis" to contact the stressful feelings associated with certain colors. Then he desensitizes his patients from these color-coded stressors.

Frenkel's technique goes something like this: while patients focus on their images in a mirror surrounded by different colored bulbs, they are asked to describe any feelings or memories that come into their awareness. Frenkel reports that old, painful memories literally "gush out" of the patients' minds during this process, frequently accompanied by the bodily symptoms associated with the original experiences. As a physician, he believes that removing stress from the mind not only reduces human disease but also unleashes human creativity. Dr. Frenkel has achieved a high degree of success in controlling anxiety, depression, phobias, migraines, suicide, computer fatigue, obesity, and drug and alcohol abuse. His work has been presented at the United Nations and will be published by Richardson and Steirman, Inc., New York, in his forthcoming book, tentatively titled *Overcoming Stress*.

ALLEVIATING PREMENSTRUAL SYNDROME (PMS)

Another very common ailment that seems to respond significantly to bright-light treatment is premenstrual syndrome (PMS). Characterized by weight gain, depression, social withdrawal, carbohydrate craving, fatigue, and irritability approximately one week prior to the onset of menstruation, these symptoms can be seriously disruptive for many women. Recently, however, Dr. Barbara Parry of San Diego, California, has shown that women treated with two hours of bright light in the evening have experienced a reversal of their PMS symptoms.[34] Although further studies are necessary, these initial results indicate that bright-light treatment may become a very effective alternative to drug therapy for PMS.

Following are one woman's feelings about the purpose of her monthly cycle:

> My menses is a time when I experience feeling "low to the ground" or "pulled to the Earth." It's as though I am being pulled into its introspective caves—to reflect on how I'm handling my immediate life experiences, now, and to listen to that stillness deep within me. It's a time when, whatever learning processes I'm in, I am enlightened and heightened with emotional awareness. I feel vulnerable, sensitive, and raw.
>
> When I busy myself with inappropriate activities not aligned with my "moon-time" callings, I feel irritable, cranky, bitchy, and drained of my vital energy. It's a cue, telling me that I'm wasting my female power and the opportunity to experience and share this opening from the Source or whatever one may call It. To me, each "moon-time" is a special gift to Woman—the gift of the "womb" and the potential of life—"Out of nothing [the Void] was created something"—whether it's my personal co-creation with the Source, procreation with my husband, or a creative project with him and others.
>
> When I nurture and listen to those inner callings, I feel peaceful and empowered. I don't always feel connected and centered. Sometimes I feel empty and void, not knowing what's going on inside, what

to do, or where to go. Yet as I honor and stay with those unknown feelings, there is a sense of stability and trust.

I often experience PMS (premenstrual syndrome) like the way I feel as the winter season approaches. I feel like my activity tempo slows down, and I feel the need to assess what I've been doing, what I've accomplished, and where I am now. When my period actually starts, I often feel like hibernating. During this hibernating period, my dreams are often lucid and powerful. I daydream a lot and feel spacey. Sometimes I feel energetic — though not the fast-paced kind. It's more like a dynamic, passive energy, where I feel very aware of reality in a big, slow-motion kind of way. By the time my period is over, I feel a sense of renewal, like in the springtime — a fresh beginning — and I go into full swing again, but with the awareness I received from my "moon-time" callings. Could a woman's cycle be a microcosm of the season's macrocosm?

In some of the Native American cultures, the woman's "moon-time" was considered a powerful time. It was through the women's "moon-time" visions that the tribal chief received guidance for his people's next move or what they needed to know as a whole. The native women were also able to coincide their menses with the new moon, believing this to be the beginning of a woman's cycle. My experience of the new moon is like the void and the "not knowing" I sometimes feel during my menses, whereas my experience of the full moon is more like the full energy I feel after my period. Were the native women attuned to a certain alignment of the moon's cycle with the woman's cycle? Could a woman's menses be, indeed, more appropriately called "moon-time," given the effect of the moon's illuminating qualities on a woman's menstrual cycle, similar to the sun's illuminating qualities on the seasons?[35]

GETTING IN TOUCH WITH LIFE CYCLES

In the particular conditions being treated or considered for treatment with bright light, such as SAD, sexual dysfunctions, and jet lag, a few questions need to be considered:

1. Which of these conditions is truly a medical disorder rather than

a symptom of something deeper that we don't understand?

2. In manipulating the body's biological clock during the treatment of shift workers or jet-lag sufferers, is the treatment truly assisting these people or is it in fact supporting their eventual "burnout"? What are the long-term effects of this?

3. Could many rhythmic disorders merely be cues to point out to us how out of touch we are with our bodies and with nature in general?

4. Is it possible that more men would experience the symptoms of SAD or even a masculine version of PMS if they weren't historically habituated to not feeling or expressing their emotions?

5. Do we judge ourselves, and are we judged by the world, for not smiling or supposedly being happy all the time? Are we really depressed, or are we just feeling our feelings? Do animals get depressed during the winter?

I have observed that many of the current medical applications of light therapy are still treating symptoms rather than causes. Even the so-called mental health practitioners are labeling most psychological difficulties as chemical imbalances. There is no question that people's body chemistry as well as their health are affected by their mental states, but to say that a chemical imbalance is the cause (rather than the effect) of a condition in most cases is a frightening diagnosis, as it supports the patient in feeling victimized and helpless rather than empowered to heal. This view only affirms that physical injury, bodily imbalance, and disease are the results of trauma, heredity, or invasion by germs, rather than recognizing that many physical afflictions are emotionally based. Instead of using light as just another drug, it is time that practitioners recognize, from their own experiences, that a more holistic application, embracing the *whole* person — mind, body, emotions, and spirit — yields much more effective results.

Those who are sensitive have always noticed seasonal shifts and the corresponding feelings they arouse. Actually, these shifts occur not just seasonally but repeat themselves on many different levels, large and small, during our lifetimes. The shifts that occur during winter and menses are truly meant for cleansing the psyche. If we don't use an opportunity for cleansing, many feelings are swept under the rug until the next opportunity arises. When unexpressed emotions are continually swept under the rug, eventual emotional and physical breakdown is inevitable. Furthermore, because of this chronic repression, certain times of the day, month, and/or seasons (for example, nighttime, menses, winter) will tend to retrigger these feelings, resulting in anxiety, depression, and general emotional upset.

I am discussing these ideas at length because with the advent of modern technology, specifically the development of the lightbulb, humans have taken advantage of Mother Nature by ignoring her laws. With respect to illumination, what began as merely an opportunity to steal a few more hours of light from Peter to pay Paul has turned into a major exploitation of ourselves and others. This has led us from an age of enlightenment to an age where we are constantly concerned about when the lights are going to go out forever. Initially we lost touch with nature and its purpose, then with those around us, and finally with ourselves. Over time this situation has created internal imbalance in the form of life-threatening diseases and external imbalance in the form of environmental destruction. Perhaps we should consider looking within ourselves for answers rather than constantly treating ourselves as the victims of some strange new disease.

There is definitely a correspondence between all things large and small. Perhaps this defines the concept of karma or describes the expression "What goes around comes around." It is as if we are a small part of a very large picture that is constantly changing — governed by an unalterable law of change. This law of change, and its correspondence to all life, was eloquently described in one of history's oldest and most highly regarded books, the I Ching. Frequently consulted by Confucius, the I Ching describes life and growth as a process of constantly changing opposite, yet complementary forces: yin/yang, feminine/masculine, contraction/expansion, ebb/flow, and so on. Understanding the law of change, which underlies everything, assists us in gaining

an awareness about life from the perspective of a participant/observer
rather than from that of a victim.

For this is wisdom:
To Love, to Live,
To take what Fate
Or the Gods may give;
Speed passion's ebb
As you greet its flow,
To have, to hold,
And in time, let go.
— AUTHOR UNKNOWN

Tolbert McCarroll sums up my feelings about this in "Seasons" from
his book *Notes From the Song of Life*:

A tree knows where it is on nature's wheel. Whatever the position — budding, in full leaf, with ripe fruit — it is all part of being
a tree.

There are seasons in your life. Do not try to escape a season. If
you try to bear fruit when it is time to bud, you may never bud.

Listen to the song of nature. Every year is a cycle. There is a time
for activity and a time for quiet. There are moments of beginning
and moments of ending. There are seasons for moving and seasons
for renewal. Be still and learn. See nature's story unfold. Watch a bird
and a tree. Learn about the commonness between you and the bird.
Let the tree help you find your place.

Be aware of the day. There are seasons to a day. The dawn is
spring. Summer is midday. The afternoon is autumn. Winter comes
at night. You were made to experience this cycle each day. Remove
your walls of protection. Move in rhythm with the day. Always
remember that tomorrow there is another cycle, another turn of
the wheel.

Every breath is a cycle of life. Take in the sweet spring of your
breath. Fill up your lungs with the summer of the cycle. Experience
the autumn joy of letting go. Be empty and still in the winter of your

breath. Now breathe again, for there is always a new beginning and a new ending.

You will never take a breath more or less important than the one you are taking now. You will never be in a day or year more or less important than the one you are in now.

Every single moment is a new beginning for all life. This present second could see the end of all. This instant is a new beginning for all. If you really jump into a now-moment you will be completely renewed.

Life, like an ocean, is made up of many waves. There are waves for each moment, each day, each year, each life. If you hunger after a sense of completeness, be in harmony with the waves.[36]

11

UV or Not UV: That Is the Question

For millions of years, life on Earth evolved under the constant influence of natural sunlight. People have always felt and recognized their connection with light. Its effects were so profoundly obvious to ancient cultures that they revered the sun as a god, blessing it daily for its gifts. Unfortunately, times have changed. As we discovered how to produce artificial light, we gradually lost our intuitive connection with natural sunlight. The sun, once considered a god, has recently been found guilty of numerous crimes and is now thought to be armed and dangerous. The public is warned: *Be cautious. Keep the sun out of your eyes, and protect yourself at all times.*

What are the real facts about sunlight? Why does the term "ultraviolet" (UV) immediately cause people to think of cancer, cataracts, aging, and wrinkles? More than 50% of the U.S. population wears prescription or sun-protective glasses made with lenses that block out most UV light. The newest plastic lenses, called UV 400, block out *all* UV light. There are even eye drops now being clinically evaluated that block out 98% of the UV light.[1] In suntan lotions, sun protection factors (SPF) 6, 10, and even 15 are no longer considered adequate protection against UV rays. SPF 25 and 30 are now recommended for *complete* protection.

This blocking of ultraviolet rays may severely weaken the body's defenses![2-4] According to photobiologist Dr. John Ott, there are strong indications that UV light through the eyes stimulates the immune

139

system. There is no question that UV light in large amounts is harmful; however, in trace amounts, as in natural sunlight, it acts, according to Ott, as a "life-supporting nutrient" that is highly beneficial. Is it possible that science has gone too far? This may be one of the biggest blunders science has made in the last fifty years.

KINDS OF ULTRAVIOLET RADIATION

Sunlight (made up of many different rays) contains large amounts of ultraviolet (UV) radiation. UV light is classified as either near-UV (UV-A), mid-UV (UV-B), or far-UV (UV-C) depending on its wavelength. Near-UV (320-380 nm), directly adjoining the violet end of the visible-light spectrum, is responsible for the tanning response in humans. Mid-UV (290-320 nm) seems to activate the synthesis of vitamin D and the absorption of calcium and other minerals. Far-UV (100-290 nm), mostly filtered out by the Earth's ozone layer, is germicidal, killing bacteria, viruses, and other infectious agents. Today, virtually all sources of ultraviolet exposure are seen as detrimental to humans. For example, all the fluorescent lights in the research laboratories of the radiological branch of the U.S. Food and Drug Administration are covered with special plastic sleeves that absorb UV light.[5] The agency does not want its employees to get a trace of the "deadly" ray.

SUN AND ULTRAVIOLET THERAPY

How is it possible that sunlight, the most powerful nutrient in our solar system, can also be so dangerous? Sun therapy was very popular in Europe from the turn of the century until the late 1930s. It was called "heliotherapy," after Helios, the Greek god of the sun.

One of the most famous practitioners of sun therapy was a medical doctor named Auguste Rollier, who was director of a sun-therapy clinic in Leysin, a town high in the Swiss Alps.[6] He attributed the therapeutic action of the sun to its invisible ultraviolet rays. Dr. Rollier, whose clinic was 5,000 feet above sea level, favored the highest mountains "because the air is transparent and easily traversed by the sun's

rays, which pass through without absorption [by the atmosphere]."
Dr. Rollier knew that his patients would get the best results if they
received the highest amount of ultraviolet light. He got such incredi-
ble results at his clinic that he published a book on this method,
La Cure de Soleil — Curing with the Sun.[7]

Tuberculosis was one of the main diseases treated by sunshine, and
many of its victims were completely cured. However, one doctor found
that the sun did not help when the patients wore sunglasses, which
blocked the healing ultraviolet light. Other conditions helped by sun
therapy included colitis, anemia, gout, cystitis, arteriosclerosis, rheumatoid arthritis, eczema, acne, herpes, lupus, sciatica, asthma, kidney
problems, and even burns.

During that same period of time, Professor George Sperti of the
University of Cincinnati was performing wonders with "tuned" ultraviolet rays.[8] Considered one of the world's authorities on UV at that
time, Sperti developed technology that could variably adjust UV rays
in order to put vitamin D in milk, tan skin, kill germs, and perform
any number of other applications. By the mid-1930s, sunbathing and
ultraviolet therapy had become known as the most effective treatments
for many infectious diseases.

In 1938, however, penicillin was discovered, and science rushed
into the new world of pharmaceuticals. Drugs became big business.
Sun therapy became as poorly thought of as snake oil and was generally forgotten except by a handful of individuals.

BENEFITS OF UV LIGHT

There is, however, another side to the story of healing with light —
and it has never been told fully. Most people don't know that there are
tremendous health benefits from ultraviolet light. Consider the
following:

1. *UV light activates the synthesis of vitamin D, which is a prerequisite
for the absorption of calcium and other minerals from the diet.*[9-13]
Robert Neer and Associates conducted a study on a group of

elderly veterans to determine if extra sunlight would increase their ability to absorb calcium from their diets.[14] All of the men received approximately 200 IU per day of vitamin D in their diets. One group of these men lived in an environment with full-spectrum lighting (which contains UV), while the other group's living quarters had ordinary indoor lighting (which contains no UV). The group that received no UV had a 25% decrease in calcium absorption while the group receiving UV had a 15% increase. In other words, the group receiving UV absorbed 40% more calcium from their diet than their counterparts who received no ultraviolet exposure.

2. *UV light lowers blood pressure.*
   It was first noticed in the early 1900s that UV radiation from the sun lowers blood pressure in both normal individuals and those with elevated blood pressure. In fact, in one study, people exposed to just one treatment of ultraviolet light noticed a dramatic lowering of their elevated blood pressure. They found that the effect lasted from five to six days.[15]

3. *UV light increases the efficiency of the heart.*
   At the Tulane School of Medicine, Dr. Raymond Johnson exposed 20 people to ultraviolet light.[16] In 18 of the 20 people tested, their cardiac output increased an average of 39%! In other words, their hearts became stronger and pumped more blood.

4. *UV light improves electrocardiogram (EKG) readings and blood profiles of individuals with atherosclerosis (hardening of the arteries).*
   In one study, 169 Russian patients with cerebral atherosclerosis received treatments with UV light.[17] A one-year follow-up indicated that all patients had an improvement in cerebral circulation, were back at work, and reported feeling better. Other studies have shown similar results.[18-20]

5. *UV light reduces cholesterol.*
   In one experiment, patients with hypertension and related circulatory problems were exposed to UV light.[21] Two hours after the first exposure, 97% of the patients had almost a 13% decrease in serum cholesterol levels. Within this group, 86% maintained

this level 24 hours later. It should also be noted that other types of fats implicated in heart disease (fatty acids, mono/di/triglycerides) are also reduced by exposure to UV radiation. This probably occurs because the body requires UV light to help break down cholesterol.

6. *UV light assists in weight loss.*
   Farm animals living outdoors don't fatten as easily as those living indoors.[22] This has also been confirmed in studies in which animals exposed to UV light lose weight. This effect is thought to be caused by the fact that UV stimulates the thyroid gland, which increases metabolism and thus burns calories. In the 1930s Swiss sun therapists found that their clients had well developed muscles and very little fat, even though they had not exercised for months. Similar conclusions are mentioned by Dr. Zane Kime in his book *Sunlight.*

7. *UV light is an effective treatment for psoriasis.*
   Reports from the National Psoriasis Foundation indicate that 80% of those suffering from this skin disease improve when they are exposed to UV light.[23]

8. *UV light is an effective treatment for many other diseases.*
   UV light has been found to be very effective in killing infectious bacteria, including several forms of tuberculosis bacteria. In 1933, F.H. Krudsen, in his book *Light Therapy*, lists approximately 165 different diseases that have been treated with UV light. The Russians and Germans routinely use UV light to combat black lung disease in miners (Russian doctors believe that the UV light helps the bloodstream to remove the dust from the workers' lungs) as well as general infectious diseases in schools and workplaces.[24-26] In other studies, patients with severe asthma have been able to breathe freely after treatment with UV light.

9. *UV light increases the level of sex hormones.*
   In a study at Boston State Hospital, Dr. Abraham Myerson found that ultraviolet light increased male hormone levels by 120%.[27] Ultraviolet light also increases the level of female hormones. Another medical laboratory found that estrogen has a sharp peak

of absorption in a portion of the UV range (290 nanometers) that many people claim is dangerous and not needed. However, this finding indicates that estrogen is *most efficient* when a woman is exposed to UV wavelengths.

10. *UV light activates an important skin hormone.*
Researchers from the University of North Carolina have shown that *solitrol* (a hormone in the skin) works in conjunction with the pineal hormone, melatonin, to control the body's responses to sunlight and darkness.[28] Solitrol, believed to be a form of vitamin D_3, works with melatonin antagonistically to generate changes in mood, circadian (24-hour) rhythms, and seasonal reproduction. Produced by the action of UV light, solitrol influences many of the body's regulatory centers as well as the immune system. The findings of these researchers might help to explain the connection between sunlight and human health.

STILL . . . IS UV BENEFICIAL OR HARMFUL?

Although these are just a few of the hundreds of medical studies done on the health *benefits* of ultraviolet light, the prevailing medical establishment continues to maintain that ultraviolet light is hazardous to our health. For millions of years, humans have evolved under sunlight, which contains ultraviolet radiation. Now, science has determined that God may have made a mistake and that *all* UV light is harmful. It is amazing how times have changed. A number of papers written early in this century talked about the health benefits of windows that transmitted ultraviolet light. In 1990, similar papers talk only about blocking ultraviolet light.

Dr. Ott is the first to agree that too much UV light is bad, but, he says, "we need a basic amount to support life and maintain a healthy immune system." He adds, "All wavelengths of sunlight are beneficial." His analogy is that giving too much oxygen at birth can blind a baby; however, he says,

> It would be foolish to jump to the conclusion that oxygen is hazardous to your health and that you should live without oxygen. Yet this

is exactly the conclusion that is drawn with ultraviolet light. If you put your hand in the furnace, it is going to get burned. But this doesn't mean you avoid heat completely and keep your house at absolute zero! The public has to understand that light is a 'nutrient' just like a vitamin or a mineral. Trace amounts of ultraviolet radiation are as important to people as trace amounts of vital nutrients.

People used to laugh at the concept that one part per million of a chemical or nutrient could have an effect on health. They thought any amount that small was virtually insignificant. Now they realize that parts per billion — and even parts per trillion — affect us. The same philosophy applies to light. When trace amounts of certain wavelengths of light are missing from your "light diet," this can have a staggering effect on your health.[29]

This is precisely the problem many people are experiencing as a result of spending most of their lives under artificial lighting.

THE PROBLEMS WITH INDOOR LIGHTS

Since sunlight (containing UV) is so beneficial to humans, there must be certain adverse effects to living and working in environments consisting totally of artificial lighting. Two important variables in this analysis are brightness level and spectral characteristics. The typical indoor environment is illuminated by approximately 600 to 700 lux, while the brightness of a summer day may reach 100,000 lux. Also, the spectral components of sunlight are vastly different from those of typical artificial lighting — the kind that exists in virtually all homes, factories, and offices.

Regular indoor incandescent light bulbs give off practically no ultraviolet light. Some companies even shield the glass to prevent the little UV that is present from coming through. One foreign company sells a "natural" light bulb that they proudly advertise emits no UV. Also, most light bulbs give off gross distortions of the visible light spectrum, emitting strong peaks of light energy in the yellow, red, and infrared portions of the spectrum. *This is highly unnatural* and is why the light in most houses looks yellowish and dingy. Dr. Ott found that wavelengths of light in the orange-pink-red range — not too far from the wavelength peaks of light bulbs — caused laboratory animals to lose their hair, show excessive calcium deposits in their hearts, and develop large, fast-growing tumors.[30] Additionally, Dr. Ott found that when animal cells were exposed to the red and infrared portions of the spectrum, their cell walls ruptured and mitosis (cell division) stopped.

Sunlight consists of a fairly balanced spectrum of color, with its energy peaking slightly in the blue-green area of the visible spectrum. Interestingly enough, blue is the wavelength most lacking in incandescent light bulbs.

Although the amount of UV emitted from fluorescent bulbs varies with each type, most fluorescent lights give off only a minute amount, which is usually absorbed by the plastic diffuser on the fixture. Another problem with all fluorescents is that they emit mercury vapor. This mercury vapor creates gross distortions of the spectrum. Dr. Ott feels that the public is being misled about this, because he believes that the mercury peaks are really *100 times* the height shown on lighting charts. He further feels that there should be a warning label with these lights saying that the mercury vapor can cause severe food allergies.

Dr. Ott also claims that there are low levels of x-rays emitted from the cathode ends of all fluorescent lights. When he placed geranium plants near the ends of the tubes, they wilted. When they were placed near the middle of the tubes, they flourished. After putting lead foil around the ends of the tubes to absorb the suspected x-rays, the geraniums placed at the ends of the tubes grew normally. He achieved similar results with bean plants.[31] Ott also claims that radio waves are emitted by all fluorescent lights. Different from the sounds heard on the radio, the radio waves given off by fluorescent lights can be detected as static when a radio is placed near a light and tuned to certain frequencies. From his observations, Dr. Ott feels that all fluorescent fixtures should be properly shielded and grounded in order to absorb the x-rays and eliminate the radio-wave emissions.

In discussing artificial lighting for indoor purposes, Dr. Ott feels that deluxe, warm-white fluorescents, which peak very close to the pink area of the spectrum, and cool-white fluorescents, which lack the blue-violet portion of the spectrum, should absolutely be avoided.

To reiterate, *ultraviolet light is a nutrient, just like a vitamin or a mineral. There really should be a recommended daily allowance (RDA) for UV light*—just as there is for vitamin C. So how, then, did sunlight and ultraviolet radiation get such a bad reputation? The public has been whipped into a level of hysteria against ultraviolet light. How can supposedly knowledgeable scientists be creating such a climate of fear?

UV STUDIES THAT CREATED A CLIMATE OF FEAR

In 1981, a study was conducted at the Medical College of Virginia in Richmond, the conclusions of which have always seemed questionable to me.[32] Monkeys were tranquilized; then their eyelids were pried open with lid clamps. With the monkeys' pupils fully dilated, researchers beamed light into their eyes from a 2,500-watt xenon lamp for sixteen minutes. This intense light contained high levels of UV radiation. *Isn't this abusive?* Although the results of the study showed that there was some retinal damage, it is hard for me to imagine that the researchers could have concluded anything else. They gave these monkeys a highly abnormal exposure to ultraviolet light *that would never happen in real life*. In real life, monkeys' pupils and eyelids *would naturally adjust* to protect their eyes, *just like the pupils and eyelids of humans do.*

Another argument science makes against ultraviolet light is that it causes cataracts. The same kinds of studies on laboratory animals concluding that UV light causes retinal damage are frequently used to conclude that UV light also causes cataracts.[33] Of course the eyes in these studies were damaged. Did they expect vision to improve? Similar studies, in which the skin of animals is repeatedly burned with high levels of UV light, also have been done to "prove" that ultraviolet light causes skin cancer.[34] Why are these scientists suggesting that ultraviolet radiation causes cancer and cataracts? Their research, which is frequently inhumane, leads to but one conclusion: *the abuse of the animals in their studies causes cancer, blindness, and death!*

There are several inherent problems with this research and, in fact, with *most* of the animal research being performed in this country. First, the sentient creatures used in these experiments are labeled "laboratory animals" in order to depersonalize them, as if their only reason for existence is for the purpose of being inhumanely experimented with and eventually slaughtered. People do terrible experiments on these animals, which are not much different from those that have been done to humans in concentration camps. Furthermore, it is impossible to come to valid scientific conclusions based on these experiments, because they are performed under extremely unnatural conditions that do not and never will exist in reality and would be considered highly abusive if they were attempted on humans. Also, when the results of these experiments are published, the researchers say, "Our research indicates that *in laboratory animals* . . . " How does this relate to humans? Is our understanding really any farther along than it was before the experiments began? Was there any time or place in history when a law was written or a supreme being told humans that it was OK for them to treat other living creatures this way? The real question is, do we need to experiment on and harm other creatures in order to learn what is and isn't good for us? As supposedly one of the most intelligent species on Earth, *shouldn't we already know these things?*

ARE WE CREATING OUR OWN BLINDNESS?

With all the current propaganda on the wearing of sunglasses with UV 400 (ultraviolet-blocking) lenses, it is possible that we are unknowingly contributing to the increased incidence of blindness and eye disease in this country. Material has come to light indicating that certain studies that have been done on the negative effects of ultraviolet light may have been based on an erroneous premise.

In a recent article entitled "Light and the Ageing Eye," Professor John Marshall of the University of London states that the body is made up of two distinct cell systems.[35] One system consists of cells that constantly renew themselves by undergoing cell division (i.e., the cornea, skin, etc.), while the other system consists of nondividing cells (i.e., the brain, retina, etc.). Organs made up of dividing cells are, we might say, constantly reborn, while organs formed from non-dividing cells maintain the same cells throughout the entire lifetime of the individual.

As an example of a nondividing cell system, Dr. Marshall refers specifically to the photoreceptors (rods and cones) and pigment epithelium cells of the retina. He suggests that certain degenerative eye diseases are probably the direct result of [what he considers to be] these nonreplenishable cells absorbing an excess amount of radiation (specifically UV) over the lifetime of the individual.

However, since light has such a profound effect on the biological functioning of the body, it must therefore also have a profound effect on the functioning of each individual cell within the body. The eye is not only a window for light energy to traverse on its way to the brain, but the components of the eye — for example, the cornea and the retina — must also be using the direct energy of light to stimulate and regulate the functioning of their cells.

In fact, 25 years ago, Dr. John Ott, working in conjunction with the research department of the Wills Eye Hospital in Philadelphia, made a sequence of time-lapse microphotographs that highlighted a previously undiscovered phenomenon. While studying the pigment epithelium cells of a rabbit's eye through different-colored filters customarily used in a phase-contrast microscope, Ott noticed that the colors of the filters used to view the cells significantly affected the biological responses within the cells themselves. Further, Ott noticed that these cells would divide only if low levels of ultraviolet radiation were projected onto them.

It thus appears clear that pigment epithelium cells *do* divide under the right conditions — which require the presence of ultraviolet radiation — and that Marshall's statements are based on an inaccurate premise. This may be due to the fact that most microscopes typically do not contain ultraviolet radiation in their light sources, nor do most laboratories have ultraviolet in their general lighting. It further appears that the typical American indoor lifestyle, coupled with our excessive use of sunglasses, might be blocking out the UV radiation necessary for normal cell-division, thus resulting in certain degenerative eye diseases, such as macular degeneration. So rather than ultraviolet radiation *contributing* to such diseases, they may instead be the result of the *lack* of it.

Is this any different than a species dying off because of an inability to reproduce? Are we creating our own blindness?

CURRENT BELIEFS ABOUT SKIN CANCER

Today, most people equate skin cancer with ultraviolet light. The two are virtually synonymous. There are certain published facts regarding UV radiation and cancer:

- Skin cancer occurs most often on those parts of the body most commonly exposed to the sun: head, neck, arms, hands.

- There is a higher incidence of skin cancer in lighter-skinned people, especially those working outdoors.

- Animal experiments have shown that larger than normal doses of UV over short periods of time are a factor in the development of skin cancer.

- It is believed that chronic overexposure to UV light, with subsequent sunburning, is a contributing factor to the development of skin cancer in 90% of the cases. As the skin is burned, free radicals are formed that are responsible not only for much of the damage involved in burning but also for the actual aging of the skin. If uncontrolled, these free radicals can cause DNA damage, which may contribute to the development of skin cancer. It should be noted that free radicals are normally kept in check by enzymes, some vitamins, and minerals.

- Skin malignancies are more prevalent in tropical and subtropical latitudes.

CHANGING BELIEFS ABOUT SKIN CANCER

On August 7, 1982, the British medical journal *Lancet* published an article that went completely against the prevailing scientific position on the relationship between skin cancer and the sun. In a study conducted at the London School of Hygiene and Tropical Medicine, England, and the University of Sydney's Melanoma Clinic, Sydney Hospital, Australia, researchers found that the incidence of malignant melanomas was considerably higher in office workers than in individuals who were regularly exposed to sunlight due to lifestyle or occupation.

One of the major researchers, Dr. Helen Shaw, found that the people who had the lowest risk of developing skin cancer were those whose main outdoor activity was sunbathing![36] Twice the risk of developing melanomas was found in office workers who had to work indoors all day under fluorescent lights. Additional research by Dr. Shaw has shown that fluorescent office lights can cause mutations in cultures of animal cells. Dr. Shaw concludes that "in both Australia and Great Britain, melanoma rates were high among professional and office workers, and lower in people working outdoors."

Further, the results of two carefully controlled studies conducted at the New York University School of Medicine confirmed the reports published by both the London School and the University of Sydney.[37],[38] Dr. F. Alan Anderson, a biophysicist with the U.S. Food and Drug Administration, believes that unshielded fluorescent lights may be responsible for approximately 5% of the total weekly dose of radiation that each person receives. In susceptible individuals, this dose may be enough to cause skin cancer.

From the above, it is apparent that the only really clear thing is that overexposure to the sun, in conjunction with certain skin types, is a major factor in the development of skin cancer. The solution then seems quite simple: moderation is the key. Mild, sensible exposure to sunlight is not only safe, it is desirable. There are people all over the world who live at high altitudes or at the equator, where levels of ultraviolet light are high, yet they are virtually free of all types of cancer. So, it is obvious that many other factors (nutrition, lifestyle, and so on) need to be evaluated.

The ultraviolet issue has been exaggerated beyond belief by people who don't wish to take responsibility for their health and well-being. Old beliefs such as boring holes in people's heads, bleeding them in times of illness, and removing their appendixes and tonsils have now shifted into a present-day wartime mentality. We have "wars" against cancer, diabetes, heart disease, AIDS, and drugs, just to name a few. People also seem to believe that these conditions are secretly planted here by outside, malicious forces, such as spies from another country or some newly discovered virus from outer space. We are being invaded — by German measles, Hong Kong flu, South American drugs, African monkeys with AIDS, and cataracts and skin cancer *caused* by the sun. Do these disorders originate in our external environment — or within us? Has anyone ever heard of the New York City disease "dirty-air-itis" or the nationwide epidemic "junk-food-cancer"? How about the child-hood disease called "good-grades-anxiety"? We've now discovered that this and other childhood disorders lead to an adult version called "getting-ahead-syndrome." Both, unfortunately, lead to heart attacks, clogged emotions, and frequently experienced heartache. We are living in a society populated by victims who are constantly at war with innocent outside sources that are only accomplices to their own self-inflicted crimes.

When will we take responsibility for the conditions of our lives and recognize that there is a consequence for every action? Isn't it our chronic impatience that creates many of our problems today? We have to have fast food, fast cars, fast suntans, and fast proof of our "scientific" theories. Once again, we need to look inside ourselves for the answers, rather than constantly pointing a finger at something "out there" that is "out to get us."

RECOMMENDATIONS

1. **Sunlight.** Spend a portion of each day (at least one hour) outdoors, regardless of the weather. Even being in the shade or on a screened porch is fine. Anything that can be accomplished outdoors should not be done indoors. Taking a walk is a nice way of spending time outdoors, while also taking time to breathe in

nature and its beauty. Unless it is an extremely sunny day that feels too bright, don't wear sunglasses, prescription glasses, contacts, or suntan lotion. Removing your glasses and contact lenses will not only allow you to receive the benefits of natural sunlight, it may also improve your natural eyesight, as long as you don't strain to see while your glasses are off. You can stay in the sun longer than an hour, but you should work up to it gradually. Don't overdo it. Avoid exposure between the hours of 10:00 a.m. and 2:00 p.m. Also, never look directly into the sun — this can damage your eyes. If you are taking a drug that reacts to light, check with your doctor before going outdoors. While indoors, sit by an open window, if possible, or at least by an unshielded closed window. This will provide you with the full visible spectrum of light (including the UV if the window is open) as well as its natural intensity, while providing a view of the outdoors — which is relaxing to both the eyes and mind.

2. **Sunglasses.** If you must wear sunglasses, consider wearing neutral gray ones. The neutral gray will reduce sunlight intensity in a balanced manner better than other available tints. Trendy colors such as pink, blue, and red are not recommended.

3. **Glasses.** If you must wear prescription glasses, ask your eye-care specialist about UV-transmitting lenses. They have to be specially ordered. These are not recommended after cataract removal. If other eye diseases exist, consult your doctor.

4. **Contact Lenses.** Tinted contacts can cause just as many problems as sunglasses, especially the new cosmetic contact lenses that come in assorted colors. They may look good, but your eyes receive highly unbalanced light. Brown and pink are the worst colors. Although the eyeglass and contact-lens industries mean well, their knowledge of light's relationship to health is minimal. Most contacts totally block the ultraviolet B part of the spectrum. Some colored contacts have a clear area in the center, but this still blocks UV light. Many contact lens, eyeglass, and sunglass wearers become light sensitive because their lenses block near-UV as well as other portions of the spectrum.

5. **UV-Transmitting Plastic Windows.** Consider installing this type of window in your home instead of regular glass. It is made of either plexiglass or acrolyte. Both of these plastics come in UVA (ultraviolet absorbing) and UVT (ultraviolet transmitting) versions. I recommend the UVT. Plexiglass is made by Rohm and Hass Plastic Company. Acrolyte is made by American Cyanamid.

6. **Suntan Lotions — Warning.** A recent report from the U.S. Food and Drug Administration concluded that fourteen out of seventeen suntan lotions containing PABA can be carcinogenic when used in the sun.[39] PABA is used in many suntan lotions to block UV radiation. Additional research indicates that PABA can cause genetic damage to the DNA in the skin. Dr. Zane Kime, author of the book *Sunlight*, firmly believes that most suntan lotions, when used in the sun, can stimulate the formation of cancer cells. He says that it is the fat in the lotions that causes the problem. My first recommendation for sunbathing is to gradually build up your time in the sun and to use no sunscreens if you have moderate to dark skin. If you must be out in the bright midday sun for more than thirty minutes, or if you have fair skin, then consider using a sunscreen that does not contain PABA.

HAS SCIENCE MADE A MISTAKE?

What does nature say about all this? The research papers don't seem to address the fact that humans evolved under natural sunlight. Are we supposed to dismiss five million years of evolution because science doesn't understand the supreme wisdom of nature? In modern times, all of a sudden, ultraviolet light is "dangerous" and should be avoided at all costs. We live in houses with no ultraviolet light. When we leave our houses, we put on our glasses, contacts, or sunglasses, which block most of the UV light. We drive in cars that also block UV light. We work all day in offices and receive no UV there either. Then at night we turn on our grossly distorted man-made lights — still no UV light.

When we finally take a break and get out in the sun, what do we do? We put on our sunglasses and cover our skin with sunscreens —

just to make sure we aren't exposed to these hazardous rays. A lot of people are now petrified to go out in the natural sunshine without some form of protection. Is there a possibility that maybe — just maybe — we have gone a little too far? Is it possible that science may have made a mistake?

> *"The most 'biologically active' part of sunlight is the ultraviolet. It is absolutely critical for optimal health."*
> —ZANE R. KIME, M.D., Swannanoa Health Report, *issues 2 & 3.*

12

Getting Well with the Rainbow Diet

In earlier chapters, I spoke of light as a nutrient for our bodies, and our eyes as the major entry points through which light profoundly affects us. In addition to the effects of ocularly perceived light on both our nervous and endocrine systems, light also affects the blood coursing through our eyes. It has been calculated that the entire volume of blood pumped by the heart circulates through the eyes *every two hours*. The eyes are the only part of the body where light can enter through a series of *transparent biological windows*. These windows — the cornea, aqueous humor, lens, and vitreous humor — allow the energy of light to directly stimulate the eyes and blood, and to indirectly stimulate all other bodily functions. How is the blood, which transports most of the body's nutrients, affected by the direct stimulation of light?

BIOLOGICAL COMBUSTION

To answer this question, it is important to first recognize that the body is a working engine, like the engine of a car. Just as a car's engine requires a balanced mixture of fuel and oxygen ignited by a spark plug, the body's engine requires a balanced mixture of fuel (nutrition) and oxygen ignited by light. In a car, the appropriate mixture of each of these components produces internal combustion, which allows the car to run efficiently. In our bodies, a similar balanced mixture of components results in biological combustion, which gives us energy to function efficiently and stay healthy.

157

It is known that every substance (vitamin, mineral, chemical, etc.) ingested by the body as food has a *maximum wavelength absorption characteristic*.[1] In other words, for any ingested substance to be fully processed or used by the body, it needs to go through a series of chemical reactions that are catalyzed (ignited) by a specific portion of the electromagnetic spectrum. Just as blue light is necessary for the proper breakdown and excretion of bilirubin in the body, and ultraviolet light is necessary for the complete synthesis of vitamin D, any substance consumed by the body requires interaction with a specific portion of the electromagnetic spectrum in order for it to be fully metabolized. Without this specific portion of the spectrum (type of light), the substance would not be fully used, resulting in some aspect of physiological functioning *being left in the dark*.

Humans appear to have the same mechanism as plants for manufacturing food. We are taught that only plants are photosynthetic — meaning they are able to use the sun directly to produce carbohydrates. Dr. Ott believes that "humans are also photosynthetic." Through our skin and eyes, we absorb light as directly as plants do. Ott says that there are *solar energy cells* all over the skin and body that help to produce carbohydrates, proteins, and DNA itself. He feels that these solar energy cells are the "Bonghan corpuscles" discovered by Korean researchers almost 30 years ago.[2] Closely related to the Langerhans cells in the pancreas, the solar energy cells are the seat of photosynthesis in humans. The light-mediated process known as photosynthesis in plants is, in my opinion, the same thing as metabolism in humans.

Although some light-activated reactions occur by way of the skin, most of them occur by way of the eyes. Light traveling through the eyes directly affects the nutrients in the blood, allowing them to be completely absorbed by the body as usable food. Without a balanced spectrum of light in our environment, we probably suffer from what Dr. Ott has appropriately called "malillumination." This condition, which is probably much more common than we would like to believe, can lead to a lack of nutritional support for certain portions of our being, resulting in chronic disease.

FROZEN LIGHT

Light, being one of our major forms of nutrition, not only affects our bodies directly but also affects us indirectly through the foods we eat. Most foods are actually light in solid form. The potency or nutritional value of light in food is directly related to the quality of the food carrying its force. The lower on the food chain we eat (i.e., the closer our food is to being manufactured directly from light), the closer we are to receiving light's full force. Eating high on the food chain (animal products) or consuming many junk, fast, frozen, irradiated, or heavily processed foods significantly reduces and/or totally eliminates light's nutritional value within that food. An example of this would be the nutritional difference between a fresh green apple and a piece of processed green candy. The most light-filled foods are probably the *blue-green algae* and organically grown fruits and vegetables. Food that has lost its light energy from overprocessing, irradiation, and so on, gradually loses its lifeforce and becomes functionally dead. Eating nutritionally dead food eventually starves our bodies, minds, and spirits, creating diminished function, frequent illness, chronic disease, and finally death itself.

As the various colors of the spectrum affect us differently, so do diversely colored foods. We first ingest the vibration of food *visually*. As we look at food, its color plays a major role in how we feel about it and how our bodies respond to it. This idea is not new, as the color of any living thing is a sign of its health. A food's color reveals aspects of its freshness and nutritional content. For example, consider how we salivate in response to certain foods we look at, even if we can't smell them or taste them. Color is not only aesthetic — it also conveys a message. Dr. Gabriel Cousens, author of *Spiritual Nutrition and The Rainbow Diet*, says that the color of a food is its signature. It is as if nature has color coded all foods so that we can intuitively and logically understand their specific purposes within our bodies.

Previously, I mentioned that the chakras, the body's main energy centers, located approximately at the sites of the major endocrine glands, are each thought to be awakened, balanced, and healed by specific vibratory energies whose visible equivalents are colors. In clinical practice, Dr. Cousens has found that a food's color has a very important psychophysiological function. Using a technique called Vascular Autonomic Signal (VAS), he discovered that different foods nourish different aspects of our being. He noticed that a food's color was directly related to the corresponding chakra of the same color and that the purpose of a particular food was to energize, balance, and heal the corresponding chakra, as well as the glands, organs, and nerve centers associated with it. In other words, each food (depending on its color) has a specific affinity for a particular energy center (chakra) within the body.

To better understand this model, refer back to the chakra chart in chapter 4 to familiarize yourself with each chakra's anatomical location, corresponding gland, personality type, and color. One side of the chart lists the Sanskrit name of each chakra and its general location, while the other side describes each chakra's corresponding gland and personality type, which are thought to be associated with certain physiological functions, personality traits, and levels of consciousness. Generally, the first three chakras (corresponding to the colors red, orange, and yellow) are associated with the physical and emotional aspects of survival, while the fourth through the seventh chakras (corresponding to the colors green, blue, indigo, and violet) represent an opening of the heart and the higher centers that nourish the spiritual aspects of higher consciousness.

Based on his research and clinical experience, Dr. Cousens recommends a "rainbow diet" of live, colorful, full-spectrum foods in order to nourish the entire being. He specifically suggests a vegetarian diet of red, orange, and yellow foods in the morning; yellow, green, and blue foods midday; and blue, indigo, violet, and golden foods in the evening. He includes foods that are gold in color because the seventh chakra (also known as the crown chakra) is frequently associated with both purple-violet and gold. He also feels that white foods (cauliflower and tofu, but not white sugar!) can be eaten at all meals, as they are considered full-spectrum. Since the progression of color in nature throughout the day moves from the red, orange, and yellow of the sunrise to the blue, indigo, and violet of the sunset, this nutritional guide aligns the daily awakening of the chakras with the daily awakening of the rest of nature.

An example of this diet might be fruits in the morning (yellow bananas, red strawberries and apples, etc.); a primarily green salad for lunch; and vegetables (eggplant, purple cabbage, beets), golden grains (wheat, rice, and millet), and legumes (purple kidney beans) for dinner. To gain a more comprehensive understanding of Dr. Cousens philosophy and nutritional recommendations, I suggest reading his book.

After many years of using light in the treatment of a wide variety of disorders, I have come to realize that one of the most powerful roles of light is the prevention of disease and the maintenance of good health. Just as we need the benefits of natural full-spectrum light, we also need natural full-spectrum food to nourish our minds, bodies, and spirits.

PART THREE

Light Years Beyond

13

A New Paradigm for Health & Healing

We have been taught that disease is caused by the invasion of germs, viruses, and so on — by "a bug that's going around." We deal with the invasion by attacking the "enemies" (germs, viruses, etc.). However, we neglect to comprehend that these so-called enemies are living *within* our bodies, and so, when we kill them, we also harm ourselves.

In reality, microorganisms don't cause diseases — *we* do. Microorganisms are merely another part of the world population trying to live in harmony with us. Their contribution to the process we call disease is only by way of our invitation. Just as ants don't think of coming into our homes unless there is food left out for them, germs don't come into our bodies unless a door is left open. That door, which opens in response to stress, holds the key to disease prevention. We don't have to focus on killing microorganisms; we merely need to change our mental, emotional, and physical environments that nutritionally feed them.

Changing our consciousness and changing our diets, lifestyles, and environments can alter the chemistry of our bodies so that infectious agents cannot survive in them and therefore are forced to leave. Human relationships are very similar. As we grow and change throughout life, some people leave our circle of relationships and other people arrive. We certainly don't have to "kill" the people we don't want in our lives anymore. Instead, clear communication that expresses our feelings and desires will usually handle the job. Thus, changing our consciousness and actions creates a very powerful effect. If our intent is to live healthful lifestyles, with respect for our feelings, bodies, and life itself, then the various aspects of our experiences — emotional, physical, and environmental — will respond so as to not create environments for disease but instead to develop stronger immune systems and increased health.

My life interest is in getting to the root causes of our afflictions. By using light to reawaken the traumatic events residing in the subconscious, these events can be brought to the conscious level and thus dealt with more effectively, in a truly deep healing, life-changing way. However, much of the therapeutic work that I've seen being practiced, even that which is called holistic, is similar to putting a Band-Aid on a cancerous tumor. At best, it only covers it temporarily. Similarly, many medical techniques merely compensate for the *effect* of a problem and rarely address the *cause* of the problem. Even many holistic approaches only *temporarily* rebalance the patients' systems until the patients once again are confronted by those aspects of their lives that originally triggered them into states of imbalance.

If healers and practitioners are not using their tools to create *deep* levels of change, then they are merely giving patients a stronger pair of crutches each year. This is often seen in the eye-care field. Patients go to typical eye-care practitioners for vision evaluations, glasses are prescribed in most cases, and the patients are told to return in a year. The following year, when their eyes have gotten worse (as is often the case), they are told that they have a progressive condition, such as near-sightedness, and that nothing can really be done. Having worked with thousands of patients over the last sixteen years, I know that this is the scenario most people experience, simply because the *root* cause of their vision problem is never looked at in the first place. Unless their practitioner is *prevention* oriented, patients are usually told that their problem is hereditary, a prognosis that doesn't support them in actively participating in their own healing process. Those patients who are brave enough to question their physicians about more holistic approaches to their specific problems are frequently made to feel foolish for even asking the question.

The typical relationship of doctor to patient in many cases violates the patient. Many doctors look upon their patients as having something wrong with them, which the doctors then think or hope they can "fix." By the same token, people have been habituated to thinking that there is something wrong with them that can only be "fixed" by their doctors. This all-too-pervasive perspective simply supports most patients in having a helpless feeling about their personal health, and it supports most doctors in their view of patients as being less than whole. I am not suggesting that doctors hide facts from their patients! However, if doctors would allow themselves to see and feel the *similarities* between their own life processes and those of their patients, they would realize that the primary experience patients want is for their physicians to *personally relate* to their situations, thus reassuring them that they *are*, and *will be*, OK. From there, treatment, whether it entails psychotherapy, medication, or whatever, becomes more effective, as the patients now are more at ease and open to deeper levels of healing. In fact, if doctors realized the power of this approach, they wouldn't have to prescribe drugs in many cases because they would be aware of the power that love, compassion, and human relationship have in the healing process.

Many physicians, as well as therapists, separate and detach themselves from their patients' processes as a way to avoid experiencing painful feelings that are *similar to those of their patients*. For instance, doctors may recommend sedatives to calm their patients. However, in reality, they unknowingly may be suppressing their patients' feelings in order to avoid dealing with their own. If a patient's fear does not surface, it will not reawaken the doctor's. Obviously, in certain cases, medication *is* appropriate. However, when the medication is used to keep one or both parties in a state of numbness, then *no real healing is taking place*.

DOCTOR, HEAL THYSELF

Being effective and powerful healers, therapists, or facilitators requires a therapeutic foundation based on personal experience, knowledge, understanding, change, and growth. To understand and effectively work with someone else's fear, anger, anxiety, sadness, physical pain, lowered performance, learning problems, poor eyesight, and so on, facilitator/healers must be able to relate to these conditions through aspects of their own personal experience. Good techniques alone are not enough! For example, assisting people with vision improvement first requires an understanding of the psychophysical aspects of how vision deteriorates. Thus, good techniques will always follow, rather than lead, the healing process.

My own personal journey has been a foundation for my understanding of how people learn, grow, and evolve. I was born in Havana, Cuba, and for the first seven years of my life spoke only Spanish. In 1955, I moved with my parents to Miami, Florida, where I experienced culture shock: I entered an English-speaking school where I didn't understand one word that anyone was saying. Although I learned to speak English within a very short period of time, academic achievement was an extremely difficult road for me. Reading did not come easily to me, and so I felt inadequate in school. This was probably the main reason that I graduated high school at the age of 19½! I was an exceptional athlete, winning numerous events, awards, and championships. However, I *felt* stupid, and my inability to read and comprehend comfortably was proof of this to me.

In 1967 I enrolled in college, only because it was the thing to do — I had no real idea of what I was studying. After only *two* years of college and a persuasive interview with an admissions officer, I applied for and was accepted into optometry school (normally four years of college is the prerequisite). The *only* reason I applied to this school was that becoming a doctor, *any* kind of doctor, was considered prestigious and usually meant that one was smart. I struggled through the first two years of optometry; however, when I began the clinical aspects of my studies I made the dean's list every quarter until graduation. I went into private practice in 1973 and, within a short time, became very successful and well known for my innovative ideas about vision improvement, learning difficulties, and other aspects of performance enhancement.

Early in 1978 I had an unexpected traumatic experience: my wife and I separated. A year and a half later we divorced. Then followed six very difficult years, filled daily with massive anxiety attacks, depression, and physical and emotional pain. During this trying period, I had two major knee surgeries. Although I had had a history of knee injuries from playing football, I recognized that part of my unconscious decision to go through with the surgery was, at that time, to make the woman to whom I had been married feel guilty for leaving me. I remember saying to myself many times, "If I could only get cancer, she would really be sorry."

Based on this experience and its painful results, I hypothesized that most diseases are diseases of the mind and that people often injure themselves as a way of bringing attention to how they feel, particularly if they are in extreme emotional pain. I refer to these years as the "fear" period of my life. I now realize that this was both the beginning of my own healing and the foundation for my understanding of human dynamics.

By mid-1984 I had emerged from this dark period. My life was in an upswing, I was doing the best work of my career, and I was feeling very satisfied. In 1986 I was awarded a second doctorate for my clinical discoveries regarding the effects of phototherapy. Even so, at the age of 38, with two doctorates and four post-doctoral fellowships, a part of me still felt "stupid." Later that year, because I wanted to be less "a doctor fixing a patient" and more "a human helping heal another human," I sold my optometric practice and decided to write a book about my clinical experiences with light therapy. For the next several months, I spent a portion of each day writing. Just when I felt I was really making progress, having written 45 pages, I suddenly lost my inspiration and could no longer continue. I shut off my computer and went on with my life.

In November 1988 I felt divinely inspired to move to Aspen, Colorado. Moving to Aspen felt as if I were *coming home*. Yet this wasn't logical — my children, friends, home, and family were in Miami. Little did I know that I was about to go into another major breakdown. As I left Miami, my earlier six-year roller coaster of pain and other emotions seemed to become compacted into the first fifteen hours of driving. My body cried and screamed as I drove, and I felt as though my life was being regurgitated from my guts. I didn't understand what was happening. The past ten years had been filled with physical pain, emotional turmoil, and some joy, but leaving Miami was extremely traumatic for me. It was leaving the womb—one minute I was part of my mother, the next minute I was alone.

This emotional trauma was soon followed by physical pain when, in early 1989, I had a severe back injury and was bedridden for three months. During this period of inactivity I had many powerful visions and awakenings, including fully reexperiencing my birth and recognizing my lack of self-love. By allowing myself to deeply feel everything, and thus give tremendous support to my healing, I emerged from this physical and emotional trauma feeling stronger and healthier, and with a powerful sense of purpose. This experience was truly a major turning point in my life. I could now understand why most of my professional career had been focused on dealing with children who had learning difficulties, assisting professional athletes with performance enhancement, and helping individuals go through major life changes. Each of their stories was my story.

Once my back had healed enough, I decided to look at the material I had written three years earlier. As I began to read my writing, I was shocked. I asked myself, Why did I write this? For whom did I write it? Would anyone be able to understand it?

I originally thought that I wanted to write my book for doctors and scientists. I wanted it to be the definitive text on the subject of light therapy. As I continued to re-read the material, though, I became more confused. It felt as though I had written it in a foreign language, and I noticed that I kept holding my breath while I was trying to figure out what I had wanted to say.

This experience reminded me of all the times in the past when I had struggled through other scientific documents and hated it. They had been so difficult to understand. At first I had been under the impression that the complexity of these documents was related to the fact that they had been written for other scientists. Although I had realized that the scientists were writing these papers for other scientists, it still had seemed to me as though the authors had been playing hide and seek with the readers without even being aware of it. At times, such documents (frequently referred to as "research") are so difficult to understand that even a bright individual frequently feels inadequate in relationship to the author, who acts as the authority.

It felt so odd. What had I gotten myself into? Throughout my life I had felt as though I wasn't smart, and now I was about to show the so-called "smart people" who was really smart. If I could write "the definitive text," then I would be looked upon as being smart, just as I had thought would occur by becoming a doctor.

For six months I struggled with the document I had previously written. I kept questioning the value of much of the information that I had originally thought to be important. What I had thought to be the "meat" of the document turned out to be the "fat." Not recognizing the value of my own intuitive insight and wisdom, I had spent most of my life trying to appear intelligent by filling my head with needless facts and forgetting that real knowledge is known "by heart" (through feelings). This was reflected in the book I had tried to write.

Every day I painfully dissected the information I had once thought to be important. Then, courageously, I excised the portions I no longer considered relevant, throwing them into the trash can on my Macintosh computer. After several months, my 45-page document dwindled down to 12 pages, which then became the beginning of this book.

After signing my publishing contract, I spent seven days per week, from eight to twelve hours per day, trying to write. The task was emotionally painful and physically exhausting. Every day was the same as the day before. I would sit, and sit, and sit, sometimes feeling empty-headed for hours. My mind would continually remind me of the statements I had heard or felt about myself many times: "You see, you really are stupid. When are you going to learn? You should be able to do this.

Everybody was right: you really are no good—you're a failure."

I was confronted by the past pain of my life and all my insecurities on a daily basis. Then a miracle happened. I noticed that if I was present with my pain long enough, something would yield; my energy would shift, and a pearl of wisdom would come through. The old expression "This, too, shall pass" began to make sense to me. The longer I sat, the more creative I became. It was like going to school all over again, only this time I was both the teacher and the student. I was beginning to understand how learning really occurs. The more I wrote, the better I felt about myself. I realized that wisdom isn't something embodied in a degree or diploma; it is the original equipment that comes with the vehicle a person calls his or her body, mind, and spirit. Unfortunately, our real wisdom is usually hidden, deeply buried by our feelings of not being enough and our need to do something, be something, or be somebody. Real wisdom takes no effort—just a lot of patience. The longer we are willing to be patient, without an investment in the "payoff," the greater the wisdom—the wisdom of self-respect.

As I contacted even deeper levels of my intuitive wisdom, I matured and realized that being "smart" was related to my ability to *feel* what was happening within myself and within the individuals with whom I worked.

BIOLOGICAL RECEPTIVITY: THE BODY'S RADAR

As a result of my own evolutionary process, and of many years of working with people, I came to the realization that everything we experience in life—physiological functions, sound, vision, speaking, hearing, and so on, consists of varying frequencies of energy that are constantly evolving. For example, EKGs and EEGs simply measure and record these frequencies and patterns of energy in our hearts and brains, respectively. The body, acting like a living radar screen, contains a multiplicity of different types of sensors that receive, record, and transmit energies. Some sensors may specifically record gross stimulations, such as the banging of a hammer or the explosion of fireworks. Others may be tuned to very subtle stimuli, such as a soft breeze or a whisper. A final group of sensors, appropriately called *ex-trasensory*, are tuned to stimuli that we neither hear nor see under normal conditions. These extrasensory sensors are probably responsible for the very sensitive, almost psychic abilities seen in many children, which seem to disappear as they become *adult-erated*. The simultaneous recording of all these different types of energy comprises that which we call *experience*.

Having discussed the ingestion of light and its subsequent effects on living organisms, I would like now to examine a specific type of energy: the energy transmitted by the body as light. It has been well documented that all living things take in and radiate light. While certain gifted psychics claim to perceive this light in the form of the body's aura, science also has documented this phenomenon. Fritz-Albert Popp, a West German chemist and physicist, found that the cells of living things radiate light.[1] These "biophotons," particles of light given off by the body, range from the ultraviolet to the infrared portions of the electromagnetic spectrum. They seem to vary in intensity depending on the specific biochemical reaction taking place, and they are most intense during cell growth.

Similar findings have also been reported by Herbert Pohl regarding the emission of weak radio signals from the cells of humans, animals, plants, and bacteria.[2] Pohl found, as Popp did, that the intensity of these radio signals was especially strong during cell division.

Interestingly, people who have experienced deep body work, such as Rolfing, often report that when sensitive areas of their body are worked on, releasing blocked energy, they literally see explosions of one or more colors in their minds. This indicates to me that when deep energy blockages within the body are released, the corresponding locked-up light energy within people is simultaneously released.

Indian scientists and physicians have found that the electromagnetic fields surrounding living things act as *identifying fingerprints* that can predict and/or identify certain physical and emotional disorders. After photographing the auras surrounding the fingertips of more than one thousand people, physicians at the Government General Hospital

in Madras, India, identified more than a dozen recognizable patterns
in patients whose conditions ranged from brain tumors to schizophrenia.[3] Although psychics routinely predict or detect disease by looking at the human aura, and although we are just beginning to validate
this phenomenon scientifically, Dinshah (one of the pioneers referred
to in chapter 6), in the 1920s, also stated that physical disease was
evident in the human aura.

All energy, whether in the form of light, sound, aroma, food, or
feelings, and so on, is in a state of flux. (The only constant is change.)
It (energy) interacts with the body through ingestion, digestion, assimilation, and excretion. If energy is obstructed or comes to a halt, it can
affect the healthy maintenance of the body, with devastating results.
Consider a river: as long as it is flowing, it is clean; however, if its flow
is obstructed and it becomes stagnant, there will be a gradual build-up
of pollution that will eventually kill all the life forms found in it.

The same is true of our emotions in our everyday experiences.
When we are in the midst of pleasurable experiences, it seems like
everything "flows" easily. When our energy is flowing so unobstructedly,
unbounded by the normal controls with which we restrain ourselves,
we often say, "Time flies when you're having fun." The physiological
expression of such fluidity is the body being healthy, like a smoothly
running engine.

Consider now that you are in the midst of a conversation with
someone, and he or she says something that is upsetting to you. Notice
what happens: you may have an emotional response — perhaps anger,
sadness, fear, or resentment; your body may start to tighten up and contract; you may eat something and experience heartburn, a stomach-
ache, and so on. It is as though the part of the experience that you are
not able to emotionally digest and assimilate is reflected by your internal organs; for example, you may not be able to physically "stomach"
your food — or your experience.

On an energetic level, our entire systems close down and contract
when we feel frightened or threatened. The digestion and assimilation
of our experiences are impaired; our energies come to a sudden halt

and get "stuck." Simultaneously, we may notice that we are holding our breaths. When we hold our breaths, our life forces do not flow. If experiences are extremely frightening, we literally hold their energy in place with our minds and bodies. This is so that later we will not have to *feel* and thus fully re-experience the pain associated with these experiences. Freud also recognized how stress affects our breathing when he said, "When our parents yell at us, we stop breathing."

On a physical level, the slowing down or stoppage of energy flow through certain portions of our bodies will cause toxic build-ups within the corresponding organs and muscles, followed by physiological dysfunction, dis-ease, and finally disease. Disease is the physical end result of a lack of energy flow through certain portions of the body's physiology.

On a mental level, those parts of the mind that record traumatic events may lock their doors to protect us from reexperiencing the pain and memories associated with these particular incidents. Since sensory recall is triggered by specific eye movements (discussed in chapter 2), fear will create a compensatory visual gaze pattern that, as a protective mechanism, restricts certain eye movements and substitutes head scanning (moving the head instead of the eyes). Over time, this restriction of fluid eye movements in certain directions of gaze results in the condition known as *astigmatism*. Although most eye doctors will say that astigmatism is usually caused by a difference in the curvature of the cornea (front of the eye), my clinical experience has shown that these curvature changes are in fact not the *cause* of most astigmatism, but the physical end *result* of a change in the way the eyes are used over time. It is obvious that our emotional responses to life affect our physical seeing.

DECREASED RECEPTIVITY

There are three factors that block biological receptivity: (1) excessive time spent under artificial light that lacks necessary wavelengths hinders stimulation of certain body sensors, which then lose a part of their function (what you don't use, you lose); (2) excessive use of sunglasses blocks certain portions of the spectrum from entering through the eyes; and (3) a trauma (emotional or physical) may cause some sensors to close down, so that they do not receive certain wavelengths of light (vibrational frequencies) even if these wavelengths are present in the light source.

Is there any significance to someone being a morning person (loving light) versus a night person (preferring less light)? Is it possible that these different types of individuals are "allergic" to the constituents of either morning light (red end of the spectrum) or evening light (blue end of the spectrum)? How about chronic sunglass wearers? Some sunglasses (yellow and pink tints) brighten things up (stimulate), some (blue and brown) dull things (depress), while others, such as neutral gray, which lies between the extremes of black and white, reduce the amount of all wavelengths of light in a more balanced manner. Is it possible that the chronic wearing of sunglasses is an unconscious attempt by the mind to "keep out" those portions of the spectrum to which people are unreceptive (which would tend to reawaken unresolved issues)?

Recently, Dr. Dhavid Cooper noticed that the eyes may selectively absorb and reflect specific wavelengths of light. This differs markedly from one person to another. In an article entitled "The Physics of Light," he wrote,

> Using my wife as a willing subject, I set up the equipment to measure directly into the pupil of her eye. Having just measured the light source composition, I knew exactly what wavelengths were being "beamed" into her eye. What was measured as being reflected back out of her eye was very interesting. Only two or three very narrow wavebands of light were being reflected back out of her eye. One in the yellow-green portion of the visible spectrum, and the other in the red end. I then did the experiment on myself, and found similar results, with the exception that only one narrow waveband, in the red end of the spectrum, was reflected out of my eye. Jacob Liberman happened to be in town, and I repeated the experiment on his eye. His results presented a very different picture than mine or my

wife's. There was a more even distribution of all wavelengths of the visible spectrum being reflected out of his eye, almost like a full-spectrum light source.[4]

The human body is like a sieve; it is built to allow energy (light) to flow through it. If our receptivity to certain aspects of vibrational experience has been reduced, then the sieve becomes clogged, impeding the flow of energy through the body and preventing the reawakening of the original experience that caused that portion of our being to close down.

By treating the body with the portion of the total spectrum that is blocked, the unstimulated sensor is reawakened. Blocked energy is loosened up, brought to the surface, and eventually dissipated. This is very similar to air bubbles being released from the Aqua-lung of a scuba diver. These bubbles have been kept in a compressed state; when they are released and allowed to surface, they dissipate as they hit the surface of the water.

State of mind determines energy assimilation, which, over time, alters brain circuitry patterns and eventually determines the state of health. Treatment with color rebalances the vibratory rhythms in the body.

Every facet of our experience is made up of energy. Early emotional traumas cause us to become unreceptive or allergic, emotionally and physiologically, to certain energetic aspects of these experiences. When we don't fully assimilate these energies, some parts of our physiological, mental, and emotional functioning remain in the dark. We can certainly remove ourselves, at least to some degree, from the allergens (situations, people, foods, etc.) that trigger our problems. However, deep healing occurs *when we become comfortable with those aspects of our experience that were previously disturbing, so that we are no longer allergic to them.* Perhaps *enlightenment* means bringing the light into those areas of our beings that we have kept in the dark. The important question is, How does the real healing take place?

HUMAN HOMEOPATHY: HOW NATURE HEALS US

It is a well-established fact that one of the most important genetically encoded programs in humans is the ability to heal ourselves. This is true of *all* life forms in nature as well. How does nature assist us in this process?

Unresolved traumatic events in life often seem to recur in various forms. It is as though we keep inviting to ourselves those situations we need in order to learn, grow, and heal. Consider the individual who was abused as a child by one or both parents. If the abusive events are never resolved and healed, this person, as an adult, creates relationship after relationship with abusive partners. Any of the current recovery/co-dependency literature can describe how common this is.

The dynamics of human relations, on an energy level, are well defined by the word *contagious*. People's emotions awaken identical feelings in those around them. For example, when a baby cries, most people in close proximity will either want to pick up the baby or have someone else pick up the baby in order to comfort it — or *so they think*. What is really going on, however, is that when a baby cries, the part of us that also wants to cry reawakens and reminds us of our own unexpressed fear and pain. Since we are taught that it is inappropriate and impolite to have and express our feelings, we usually pick up the baby and give it a breast or a bottle in order to suppress *its* feelings. What we often don't comprehend is that *we are doing this for ourselves, not for the baby*.

Adults who express and release painful feelings seem to trigger uncomfortable responses in most of the people around them. For reasons that are usually dormant, bystanders have a need to take care of "feeling" people by comforting them and reassuring them that their feelings will pass. What the "caretakers" don't realize is that *the only thing that they really want to do is suppress the other people's pain* so that they won't have to confront their own. If, instead, the feeling people were *supported* in expressing and releasing their feelings, which is something nature intends, the growth and development of *everyone involved* would actually be enhanced. When the feelings of others reawaken our own unresolved feelings, it gives us the opportunity to become aware of the parts of us that need healing. By using these sometimes painful experiences opportunistically, we expand our awareness and nourish our evolvement, just as rich fertilizer assists the growth of a plant.

Our inability to express our feelings stems from the fact that we have been taught how to speak but not how to listen — either to ourselves or to others. For example, how many times have you started formulating a response to someone's communication before they finish making it? And how often do you respond without really *feeling* your response to the other person's communication? If you pretend not to see, hear, or feel what you actually see, hear, or feel, then the portions of your being that are responsible for processing this information will eventually begin to malfunction. Perhaps this is the reason why we develop poor eyesight, auditory impairment, and emotional rigor mortis.

Nature provides us with just what we need to assist us in the process of growth and development. There is an old Latin expression, *Similia similibus curentur,* meaning "Let likes be treated by likes." In other words, those aspects of life to which we are unreceptive *are probably just the medicine we need to ingest* to assist us in healing our reactivity to the unreceptive situations. Such medicine will thus expand our awareness. This universal law of cure, referred to as the Law of Similars by Hippocrates and Paracelsus, became the basis of the modern science of homeopathy. Formulated by German physician and pharmacist Samuel Hahnemann in 1810, homeopathy treats the whole person rather than just the disease.[5-6] Hahnemann's contention was that physical disease is, in essence, a disturbance in the body's vital force.

Another very important concept in homeopathy, which was introduced by Hering, is that *healing begins in the deepest parts of our beings* — the emotional/mental levels — and then spreads outward to the physical level.[7] Homeopathy views *symptoms* as the efforts made by an organism to defend and heal itself. A basic premise in homeopathy is that the most appropriate remedy for a patient is one with a *vibration* that is *equivalent* to the patient's pathology. Furthermore, the more dilute the remedy, the greater is its potency — that is, *less is more*.

It appears that many of homeopathy's basic principles are patterned after nature's methods of healing. These principles affirm my own clinical observations and indicate the following:

1. The mind and body are interconnected, thus creating a cycle in which each continually influences the other, so that both affect the development and remediation of mental and physical disorders.

2. Although many aspects of behavior, personality, and appearance are learned attempts to cope with the environment and assist in healing, many aspects are also deeply rooted in our constitutional types, thus creating automatic reflexlike reactions to different conditions and situations.

3. To heal our basic dysfunction or disease, we must be treated with a remedy that vibrationally matches all of our symptoms. Other people or situations with issues that are similar or complementary to ours will trigger the particular emotional/physical issues within us that we are attempting to heal. This is one way in which our species evolves.

4. The subtler the remedy, the more potent it is.

5. During the process of healing, deep emotional issues will usually surface first, followed by their physical counterparts.

The effectiveness of homeopathy as a natural medical treatment suggests that we may in fact be *each other's* homeopathic remedies, and that the *gentler* we are with each other, the greater our healing will be. What I am suggesting is that those incidents in our lives that most trigger our feelings are really bringing our awareness to the very sensitive, wounded, and usually armored portions of our beings that most need healing. This is nature's way of bringing subconscious information to the conscious level so that we can effectively deal with it.

When nature provides us with an opportunity for growth through the triggering of our sensitive feelings by other people or situations, most of us, due to our cultural conditioning, avoid our *true* feelings and instead develop and act out addictive patterns. The baby in the earlier example attempts to express its feelings, but someone shoves a bottle, nipple, or pacifier into its mouth. The message received by the baby is: *when feelings arise, the appropriate way to deal with them is to put something in your mouth.* In adults, this results in overeating, smoking, abusing drugs and alcohol, and so on. In other words, what we don't address, we suppress.

"Neurosis is always a substitute for legitimate suffering."
— Carl Jung

"Grieving is the healing feeling."
— John Bradshaw

"The gain is in proportion to the pain" [a popular proverb in ancient times!].
— Verse 26, chapter 5, Ethics of the Fathers, The Talmud

14

Becoming Illuminated with Light

"The significant problems we have cannot be solved at the same level of thinking we were at when we created them."
— ALBERT EINSTEIN

So far I have described light as a tool to treat different functional and pathological conditions. However, light is also a tool to expand our awareness of emotional and mental patterns so that we can create an internal environment where vibrant health is the norm.

WHAT I WAS TAUGHT

My first course in light therapy (called Syntonics) was based on the work of Dr. Harry Riley Spitler, who had developed a rather elaborate course. However, by the time I was introduced to the work it had been trimmed down to a simple, almost cookbook-style approach. Spitler differentiated people according to body type, creating approximately twenty different color-filter combinations that were commonly used for treatment. Present-day Syntonics practitioners, however, do not utilize body typing, and they have reduced the number of commonly used filters to approximately five. A major premise of the syntonic approach is that most dysfunctions are the result of an imbalance between the sympathetic and the parasympathetic portions of the autonomic nervous system. Filters are separated into three categories according to their effect on the autonomic nervous system: (1) those that stimulate the sympathetic nervous system, (2) those that stimulate the parasympathetic nervous system, and (3) those that act as physiological or emotional equilibrators.

For example, the yellow-green filter, considered a physiological equilibrator, is recommended in all cases in which a chronic imbalance or disease exists, such as those involving a head trauma that occurred several years prior. Blue-green is also considered a physiological equilibrator; however, it is recommended in cases that are acute or of recent origin, such as fevers and inflammations. Magenta (a combination of red and violet) is considered an emotional stabilizer and is used in cases in which an emotional component appears to be present.

Spitler's original model, based on medical theories of the 1920s, viewed dysfunctions and diseases primarily as imbalances in the body's physiology or the results of trauma. The idea that emotional issues might underlie many physiological imbalances was not considered to any great degree. In those days, one's problems had to be severe to be considered emotional in nature. Minor emotional issues were usually swept under the rug and not expressed, which was the norm of the period.

HOW WELL SYNTONICS WORKED

In my own practice, the clinical application of Syntonics in some ways seemed simplistic. However, the treatments were very effective, often producing miraculous results in short periods of time, as can be seen from the cases discussed in chapter 7. Although these particular cases may seem sensational, I achieved similar results quite often, particularly with children, whom I found to be more receptive to change than adults.

Functioning as an optometrist, I used Syntonics to treat an entire array of vision problems (crossed eyes, nearsightedness, visual discomfort, etc.) as well as vision-related learning problems (reading difficulties, poor attention span, etc.). However, the question that arose repeatedly in my mind was, What are the underlying issues causing these dysfunctions? Based on the results I was achieving clinically, it became obvious to me that not all cases of crossed eyes or nearsightedness were hereditary; in fact, I found that most of them were *not* hereditary, nor were learning problems mostly secondary to neurological dysfunctions, as was the popular belief. Other questions that constantly puzzled me were, How could a specific filter combination such as magenta (an emotional stabilizer) affect everyone in the same way? Does any one thing affect all, or even most, people the same way? Is it really possible for a patient's emotional issues to be healed without the patient recontacting the original cause of his or her imbalance? How was I handling and resolving the emotional traumas in my own life? I had to look deeper within my own experience!

EXPLORING THE UNEXPLORED

As I worked with more and more patients, I began to realize that the so-called "rules" about the effects of various filters were applicable only in certain cases. For example, while magenta did in fact calm many patients, its effects were disturbing to others. This is similar to the difference in nutritional value received by people eating exactly the same meal or to how differently people respond to a particular situation or person. Do all of us taking the same vitamins receive the same benefits?

It soon became very clear to me that the effect of any therapy was specifically related to the biological *receptivity* and psychic make-up of the person being treated and that so-called absolute rules were not applicable to everyone. I also realized that an important aspect of any form of treatment is its purpose. Is the intention to palliate the problem (make it less severe without curing it), to compensate for the problem (such as recommending eyeglasses for a nearsighted person), to rebalance the patient (a temporary solution), or to get right to the heart of the issue? From both my own experiences and those of my patients, I realized that there was no way to avoid or skim over deep emotional traumas from the past that were often at the root of current issues. Trimming the tops of weeds only stimulates them to grow back faster. Pulling them out by the roots is the only solution. Uncovering and unearthing the deep issues of our lives is not an easy task, as these issues are usually deeply embedded, well protected, and masterfully camouflaged under many layers of disguise.

THE TIP OF THE ICEBERG

Imagine being on an ocean liner. As you look off into the distance, you notice a large iceberg. Although what you *think* you see is the iceberg, what you really see is only its tip. It is the portion of the iceberg under the water's surface that can be injurious to the hull of your ship. This is a perfect example of how "what you see is *not* what you get." Icebergs are nature's example of the relationship of the conscious mind to the subconscious mind. It is estimated that the portion of an iceberg above water is only 10% to 12% of its total mass. Interestingly enough, the conscious mind is the same percentage of the total mind. Most people's lives are run by the mass below the surface.

The task is to bring the subconscious up to the conscious level. If we could uncover the issues under the surface that govern our lives, we could then acquaint ourselves with these issues, work with them gently, and finally befriend them. It is like slowly taking off the leaves of an artichoke and eventually getting to its heart—the core of its being. Since all of our external expressions in the world are related to matters within our hearts, gently rebonding with our hearts can affect every aspect of our functioning and being.

COLOR SENSITIVITY

After a bit of time in my practice, I began developing a subjective color-preference technique. What I found was that if I gave patients a choice between two opposite colors (such as red and blue), they always instinctively seemed to prefer one color over the other. When I started each session, I explained to the patients that I would call out pairs of colors and that the ones with which they felt most comfortable would immediately appear in their minds—since their bodies understood what I was looking for, they would respond intuitively without any thought.

While using these pairs of colors (red and blue, yellow and violet, and lime and turquoise), I noticed some interesting responses. When I compared patients' subjective preferences to what I intuitively felt they needed, they were almost always the opposite. For example, if they preferred blue to red, in most cases red was the color I felt they needed for deep healing. It seemed as though the colors they felt most comfortable with or soothed by were just the opposite of what I felt they needed. It reminded me of the fact that most people in life are comfortable with avoiding things that are in any way disturbing.

Recognizing that everyone perceives color differently, I decided to have people look directly at light of different colors and respond that way. After doing this with hundreds of patients, I noticed that people were receptive or unreceptive to specific colors in varying degrees. Some colors brought on feelings of ecstasy while others immediately incited anxiety attacks, with associated physical symptoms.

For example, a patient with a headache might find that a certain color reduced the pain or totally eliminated it, while another color exacerbated it. I questioned what the difference was between treating someone with colors to which they were receptive (comfortable with) versus colors to which they were unreceptive (uncomfortable with). I wasn't as concerned with the colors people felt comfortable with as I was with the colors that disturbed them. The disturbing colors seemed to represent, or in some way be related to, painful experiences in patients' lives, whether these experiences were recent or long ago.

DEVELOPING NEW METHODS

Determining the most effective way to utilize color in working with people caused me to once again reexamine the basic tenet of homeopathy that states that *the most appropriate remedy for a patient is one with a vibration that is equivalent to the patient's pathology*. In other words, the color or colors that exacerbate the problem are perhaps the ones to treat with! During that same period of time, it was brought to my attention that during the 1930s and 1940s, Royal R. Rife, a pioneering scientist, developed a microscope that could determine the exact "color" associated with a particular virus or other infectious microorganism.[1] He found that irradiating the organism with the same color of light it gave off would very quickly destroy it.

At this point I noticed that the behavior of patients with addictive personalities became more addictive or less addictive depending on the colors at which they looked. For example, an alcoholic would look at one of the colors to which he was receptive (comfortable with) and be fine; a color to which he was slightly unreceptive might elicit an urge for him to drink juice or soda; a color with which he was most uncomfortable would cause him to want to drink alcohol. It was now becoming clear to me that when situations in life trigger fear or discomfort, our inability to be present with these feelings as well as to deal with them forces us to protect ourselves by avoiding, or *numbing out*, the situations and going into an addictive behavior pattern.

Such a behavior pattern may be totally unconscious. For instance, the body may know that the energy content of a particular food, such as chocolate, or a particular drink, such as vodka, when combined with the energy content of fear may temporarily alleviate that fear. *This, I believe, is the basis of all addiction.*

Since the degree of receptivity varied from color to color for each patient, I eventually decided to arrange the colors for treatment from least unreceptive (least uncomfortable) to most unreceptive (most uncomfortable). Starting the treatment with a color that was only mildly uncomfortable allowed patients to gradually develop an authentic security in their ability to go through this process. This would then transfer to their ability to handle stressful situations in their lives. In addition, I wanted to establish a trusting relationship between myself and these patients so that they would feel comfortable working with me, especially as deeper and more painful issues began to surface. Matters of the heart cannot be attacked with a machete; rather, they must be handled with love and compassion.

When I first began using this approach, there were some interesting responses from patients. Some began grieving as old painful events, in the form of lucid dreams or vivid flashbacks, surfaced. One young lady, in the midst of her eleventh treatment session, re-experienced being raped. Although her pain was extreme, she eventually came to terms with the situation and realized that this powerful issue in her life was getting in the way of her ability to have intimate relationships with men.

Many of my colleagues thought my approach was crazy. They were frightened by any possibility that *their* treatment might disturb a patient. Nonetheless, my own process of deep inner growth — particularly allowing myself to feel my own pain in the presence of another human being — was the impetus that kept me moving forward with this approach. I was now beginning to understand the process by which we heal. Although the technology of phototherapy is, in itself, very powerful, its true power blossoms only when the awarenesses that it stimulates can be expressed in the presence of a loving, compassionate human being. In other words, the interaction between the patient and the facilitator is primary.

From very early in our lives, most of us have wanted to be with people who would allow us to be exactly who we are, rather than love us only conditionally — that is, when we are cute, smart, or well behaved. I discovered that treating patients by way of their eyes (the windows of the soul) with colors to which they were not receptive and that were in a specific sequence would reawaken old and unresolved emotional issues that seemed to be at the core of the physical dysfunctions they were experiencing.

COLOR RECEPTIVITY AND THE CHAKRAS

One of my most important clinical discoveries was that the colors to which people were unreceptive correlated almost 100% of the time with the portions of their bodies (described by the chakra chart in chapter 4) where they housed stress, developed disease, or had injured themselves. For example, a person might be uncomfortable looking at the color blue, and during the case history I would discover that this person had chronic sore throats, significant dental problems, difficulty with verbal expression (a function of the throat and mouth), and had had his or her tonsils removed.

Additionally, I noticed that once patients had resolved the emotionally painful issues triggered by the colors, then looking at these colors, which was originally uncomfortable, actually stimulated feelings of joy and euphoria.

THE CASE OF NANCY

Nancy, a 47-year-old woman, experienced a nervous breakdown at the age of 45. In the four years prior to that, both of her parents as well as her husband's father had passed away. The subsequent relationships with her four siblings became awkward. Old resentments that had never been expressed began to surface, with ensuing power struggles, false accusations, and nasty letters. All of this resulted in difficult communications and tremendous pain for Nancy and her siblings. She went into a deep depression, feeling possessed by a relentless inner dialogue of overwhelming rage and intense self-hatred.

Nancy first went to a psychiatrist who wanted to put her on medication. She refused to take antidepressants, feeling that they were just another way of numbing out her problems. Her psychiatrist's approach was to try to get her to disassociate and distance herself from the people whom she felt were holding her in pain. Feeling that this was not the approach she wanted, she went to another psychiatrist who focused on the mental/theoretical aspects of what was happening. Again, she felt that this was not helping her to resolve the tremendous hate and resentment she was feeling. During this time she developed arthritic-type symptoms — painful aching in her arms, legs, and hips — as well as an irregular menstrual cycle.

She saw specialists of all kinds, including general practitioners, gynecologists, arthritis specialists, a Lyme tick disease specialist, acupuncturists, a chiropractor, and an orthopedist. Diagnoses included uterine cancer, adrenal problems, Lyme tick disease, rheumatoid arthritis, tennis elbow, depression, a hormonal imbalance secondary to menopause, and finally a verdict of "it's all in your head." She underwent numerous tests, biopsies, x-rays, and blood work-ups. All were negative, but her pain persisted. It seemed that no one could help her.

Nancy began reading self-help books, going to retreats at a nearby monastery, and doing a lot of writing; however, she still felt paralyzed by her physical pain and mental depression. At this point she attended one of my lectures and, although skeptical, was drawn to my approach and came in for an initial session.

I felt that her physical problems were primarily caused by unresolved emotional issues and told her that she would need to address *both* simultaneously if she expected to get well. I also referred her to a local internist whose holistic approach would support her healing. He recommended that she alter her diet and eliminate foods that might be aggravating her condition.

Several other aspects of Nancy's medical history came out during her first visit with me. She was very nearsighted (20/200 in her right eye, and 20/300 in her left, without glasses). She complained of constant discomfort in her eyes, an inability to read for any length of time, and trouble adjusting to her bifocals. She also had had three eye-muscle surgeries to try to correct an eye that had been turned outward since she was very young. It was obvious to me that the surgeries were unsuccessful, as one of her eyes was constantly drifting out and up toward the side. She was totally addicted to her glasses, and the thought of taking them off, even for short periods of time, frightened and angered her. During that initial visit, I observed that Nancy's physical pain worsened when she gazed at certain colors and improved when she looked at others. I also noticed that her field of vision was much smaller than normal, especially in her left eye, which was the one that turned out.

Nancy lived approximately 40 minutes from my office, so, rather than have her come in daily, I scheduled her to come in once a week. I also recommended that she perform *daily* phototherapy self-treatments at her home with a device that I lent her. On her first visit, she said, "My arms feel as if they have tourniquets tied tightly around them at the elbows." Feeling constant pain day and night, Nancy wondered if she would ever have any relief. I told her that her symptoms would probably worsen before they got better, as treatment meant going right to the heart of her problem. At this point she had no idea what I really meant by that but decided to go ahead with my recommendations.

We began treatment with a combination of yellow-green and red-yellow light, which caused her pain to worsen, indicating to me that we had touched on a sensitive area. I had to keep reminding her that in order to see the light at the end of the tunnel, she first would have to walk through the tunnel. My treatment was not designed to make her "feel good"; rather, it was designed to bring to the surface those unresolved life issues that I felt were the real cause of her physical ailments. I was certain that there was something she did not want to "look at" and was sure that it would be only a matter of time before it would surface. The only question in my mind was whether she would be willing to go through the process.

We continued with these same colors until they no longer irritated her and then started on a combination of turquoise and indigo light for ten minutes each, twice a day. Although the turquoise was not very stressful for her, the indigo triggered strong reactions, followed by significant changes. Her initial reactions included feeling even more irritable and angry than she had with the prior colors, frequent "flying off the handle" and crying (which did not seem related to anything specifically going on), and occasional panic attacks. These feelings were familiar to Nancy, as they reminded her of her previous break-down. Old nightmares of the past and dreams of anxiety started surfacing, as well as feelings of irritability and anger at why the treatment was not improving her condition. One of her nightmares involved chopping up one of her siblings. She once again felt paralyzed by fear. She didn't think she could stand to go through these feelings all over again.

At this point Nancy began discussing with me the sexual abuse she had experienced as a child and the inability she had felt to express her need for help at that time. She had felt that she could not possibly tell her father that *his* own father had been sexually abusing her for a couple of years. It now became clear to me why she had become near-sighted during that period of her life. This was obviously a situation she couldn't bear to look at. If this experience could be brought out of the closet and openly looked at, perhaps the mental grip that was partially paralyzing her vision could be released. How would this affect her physical eyesight?

Although the results of a recent eye examination had suggested an even stronger prescription than her current one, I recommended that Nancy get a second pair of glasses with a 20% *reduction* in strength from her current glasses and that she wear these occasionally instead of her normal glasses. Additionally, I recommended some vision therapy to improve her ability to use her eyes as a team. During the process of learning the exercises, she suddenly had a moment of clear vision *without* her glasses. This immediately brought on a severe anxiety attack, debilitating her for the next 45 minutes. Her fear was so intense that she literally fell on the floor and began to shiver. I covered her with a jacket and spent the balance of the session sitting on the floor with her, emotionally supporting her as she felt her pain and expressed her feelings. Although this experience was very frightening for her, I shared with her my own many similar experiences, which helped her to feel comfortable about letting her feelings out and to feel secure in the knowledge that she would survive. She knew she wasn't alone.

Although the adjustment to her new glasses was initially very difficult, within two weeks Nancy was wearing the weaker glasses full time and noticed that her eyes felt more comfortable, even while driving her car.

One morning at her home, after twenty minutes of indigo treatment, she started screaming and crying, feeling totally out of control. For about fifteen minutes she couldn't tolerate the sensations of touching, tasting, hearing, smelling or looking at anything. She felt overwhelmed by her senses. At this point her husband called me, very concerned about whether she should continue treatment. Having seen this kind of response many times previously (especially in *myself*), I realized that as long as her symptoms were being exaggerated, we were on the right track. *A major key to getting well is becoming comfortable with those aspects of our lives that were previously uncomfortable.*

The more Nancy worked with the indigo light, the more she noticed a shift in her experience and perspective. Three weeks following the morning of hysteria, she wrote the following passage in her journal:

> I can't believe it, but lately I am waking up in tears of joy and euphoria, with an incredible sense of peace, which carries into the day . . . the indigo light symbolizes to me a light within myself — a light that has been patiently waiting within me — lately in the mere gasp of a flicker — not quite able to penetrate so much darkness but a light now burning brighter and starting to melt my heart. . . . I am filled with love and gratitude.

Nancy felt that she was starting to come alive again. Her attitude shifted from one of "I *should* or *have to* go through this process" to one of "I want to — I like to — I have the energy to do this." She also said,

> My physical pain was trying its best to lift out of me. I was getting the feeling that it didn't want or need to be with me anymore, but on the other hand that it didn't exactly know how to leave. I mean, after all, I was giving it an awfully good home and had locked the door tight on it. My aches and pains have substantially decreased . . . by as much as 85%.

She also noticed that when her pain resurfaced, it was usually during times of stress. She was slowly changing in her ability to look at her pain and embrace it, rather than ignore it, fear it, or treat it like an enemy.

After approximately three months of treatment, I found that Nancy's ability to see without her glasses had now improved from her original 20/200 with both eyes open to approximately 20/40. Based on this, I once again recommended a reduction in her eyeglass prescription — this time to a prescription 50% as strong as her original one (the reduction in eyeglass prescription usually doesn't correlate exactly with the degree of eyesight improvement). After struggling with this new pair of glasses for about two weeks, she discovered that she saw better with them than with her previous glasses. At this point she threw out her old bifocals and found that she could read a book without any glasses at all. Her previous feelings of disorientation, difficulty in hearing, and panic when she wasn't wearing her glasses had now disappeared. She commented that she had never felt so much joy and energy in her life:

> I have learned in this brief time that joy and happiness, and even serendipity, do not necessarily come only in brief little fleeting moments — there are long, sustaining stretches to be experienced. I know, because it is happening for me. And to think that just two and a half years ago I was overwhelmed by a depression that I thought would never lift. Ultimately this is a spiritual journey — an experience of increasing Grace. An experience of the heart — not of the mind.

Nancy and I continue to work together and are making wonderful progress. Reaffirming her experience of embracing and befriending her fear and pain are the following suggestions by the channeled entity Bartholomew, from his book *I Come As A Brother*:

> The moment you sense that painful feeling within you, say to yourself, *"I love this feeling.* I welcome it. It doesn't have to go anywhere or change. It is part of me. I accept this feeling." And the warmth which is always there, moves over to this "rock" and begins to smooth it, surround it, and make it porous. So out of the power of your love for this "rock," "it" takes on the power of your love. It becomes filled with your love! Love pours through this "unlovely" feeling-mass, surrounds it, uplifts it, and it becomes "lovely." And you find you are capable of holding two things: *your love and that agony.* Your love is so vast that there is nothing that it will not hold, and using that vastness is what you've got to learn. No grief is so great that you cannot hold it within you and also hold the vast power of your love at the same time. You do not have to choose. You can have all the grief, you can have all the illness, you can have all the sorrow, all the regrets, all the guilt, and there is no need to worry because all the love in your heart is so vast it will hold anything. These emotions are your children. *They are your children!* All they want is your love. You have created them, and then you treat them like bastards. But you created them! When you warm these emotions through your love

of them, through your acceptence of them, then the words "trans-
mutation" and "transformation" become real. Once you decide that
you are so vast that you can hold anything, you will be fearless —
fearless because you have learned there is nothing that can come to
you from this world that you cannot hold. There is no grief so great,
no event so horrible that you cannot hold it in you, smooth it, warm
it, open to it, and love it. Those of you who have had traumatic
beginnings, don't run. Love them. Don't try to love the people,
please. Love the feelings.[2]

In Nancy's case, the colors to which she was most unreceptive were
the red-oranges and the blue-indigos. Red-orange relates to the chakras
associated with survival and sexuality, whereas blue-indigo relates to
the chakras (throat and pituitary) associated with expression and seeing on the physical level. The early trauma to her eyes (three eye
surgeries), combined with her experiences of sexual abuse, which she
did not want to look at (a function of her eyes) and, because of her
fear, could not express (a function of the throat), caused those portions
of her body to close down. In treatment, these specific colors did in
fact bring up the associated memories, and her physical healing in
these areas was dramatic.

KAY: A MIRACLE STORY

In 1989, Kay, a 41-year-old therapist with a background in emer-
gency medicine, came into my office for phototherapy, intent on halt-
ing the progressive deterioration of her eyesight. She was wearing
bifocals, and without her glasses could focus clearly only a couple of
inches from her nose.

Although Kay came in for vision improvement, it became obvious
from her personal and medical history that she had been born into a
severely dysfunctional family. Most of her life had been spent in emotional and physical breakdown.

Kay's mother had been a talented artist who for years had experienced wide and variable mood swings on a daily basis, followed by
periods of deep depression. Her condition had finally been diagnosed

as paranoid schizophrenia. In addition, her mother had suffered from a severe rheumatic heart condition for 33 years. Fearful, temperamental, and prone to rage attacks, she had frequently said to Kay, "It is such a pity you were born a girl." Her mother had herself been severely abused, neglected, and abandoned as a child. She had married a man who hated women and who had thrown her out of the house when Kay was eleven years old. Two years later her mother had committed suicide.

Kay's father had grown up taking care of his five younger siblings as well as the emotional needs of his extremely young mother. He consequently developed a hatred for women and children. This hatred, along with his training as a career military officer, had led him to treat Kay as a slave, frequently reminding her that "all women are born lazy, are no good" and that he wasn't going to permit dishonesty and freeloading in his house. He had forced her to scrub the walls, floors, and corners of the house with a toothbrush. Sitting down or reading was not allowed. She remembers, "Every interaction with him was demeaning and humiliating. I hadn't done anything wrong, except be born."

When her mother had committed suicide, Kay had been told by her father, "I want you to behave. Do you hear me? I don't want to hear a peep out of you, and if you ever mention that person's name again, you'll have me to answer to!" In remembering this incident during treatment, she recalled, "Forbidden to cry, my asthma and severe allergies started . . . I had failed to save my mother, when all she ever asked of me was to save her from Dad. I thought I had deserted her."

For the five years prior to my treatments, Kay had been visiting her physician every two weeks because of a collapsed immune system. She was receiving spleen extract injections three to four times per week, megavitamins, imipramine hydrochloride (an antidepressant), and homeopathic remedies. She couldn't take antibiotics due to the fact that she had taken so many during her life that they now had little or no effect on her. She suffered from chronic sinus infections, severe chronic bronchitis, and asthma. At the age of 24, Kay had had a hysterectomy and soon after developed endometriosis (an infection of the uterine mucous membrane) and fibrocystic disease of the breast. Her lungs had been functionally crippled from chemical pneumonitis since 1982. During the summer of 1988 she had been told that she needed a bilateral mastectomy. She had also recently undergone significant lower back surgery for a degenerative disk disease that had caused her severe pain for many years. The state of Colorado classified her as disabled.

During her light treatment, Kay frequently found that old memories surfaced. Certain colors, expecially red and yellow, triggered severe anxiety and physical symptoms such as headaches, nausea, and asthma that were associated with flashbacks of frightening experiences. She also experienced full recall of events in her life that she had completely forgotten or that she had remembered only in fragments. For example, she remembered and relived an experience, when she was eight, of being kicked by her mother across the linoleum floor of the kitchen into the base of the stove:

> It was strange watching Mom hurt me with the handle of a wooden spoon from the vantage point of looking down on the scene. I then relived Mom looking at my body, shaking her head as if to clear it, and leaving me unconscious and bleeding, covered only with crawling flies. I next relived being lowered into the pink bathtub while hearing, "If you tell anyone, I'll kill you." I now know why I have always panicked if a buzzing fly got into my house. I had blocked the entire incident, but it fit with the feelings of terror, confusion, horror, and shame I have carried most of my life.

Kay also remembered childhood experiences surrounding the deterioration of her eyes. She had difficulties in school with math, reading, and spelling, and hadn't been able to see the blackboard from the first row. She actually remembered being told that she was slow and lazy, and that "if you would just apply yourself, you wouldn't have to always look so stupid." From these experiences, she became frantic:

> My mind had stopped working. Was I becoming just as crazy and

worthless as Mom? I didn't know what was happening. I just knew I couldn't trust my mind, or my eyes, to function correctly, so I deserved to be humiliated and punished by Mom, Dad, my teachers, and other students.

I can see now that my secret knowledge of Mom's adultery with my math teacher affected me deeply. I didn't have permission from my family to share my confusion with anyone. The knowledge just went underground. I wasn't supposed to *see* what was going on, so I suddenly couldn't see. I wasn't supposed to *know* what was going on, so I suddenly couldn't read or think clearly. Parents made the rules. The rules were to be obeyed. What parents did was right. What parents did was good . . . so I reasoned emotionally that because I felt so bad I must be the one who was bad . . . I internalized and personalized my mother's behavior; I needed to be punished for feeling bad and doubting my mother's explanations.

During another light treatment, I relived riding my bike. It was a hot day. My hair was in a pony tail. . . . When I got home, I ran into the house quickly, to change and get to my chores. But when I pulled the shirt over my head, I felt and heard the angry buzzing of a wasp. I screamed, but it was too late. I was stung eight times down my spine. Mom came down the hall. She was furious, and began pounding me to my knees, saying, "How dare you scream like that? Who do you think you are to startle me? I'm going to teach you a lesson you'll never forget."

So she hit me over the head and shoulders with her fists, and kicked me as I tried to hold onto the side of the bed. I couldn't catch my breath. I was wheezing, so she beat me harder to make me shut up and stop making such awful noises. Then she had her hands around my throat to throttle me into silence. . . . She then left the house looking disgusted. I was left wheezing and nearly unconscious on the bedroom floor.

As a teenager, Kay had become a super-responsible overachiever in an attempt to earn her father's love. She had driven herself without mercy, becoming a National Honor Society scholar in spite of her dyslexia. Married at nineteen, she had entered into another dysfunctional relationship with her new husband, which had ended in divorce two years later. Her son had then become her life and joy until he had choked on a piece of candied apple while playing with his puppy and had died. She had become numb with grief for the next year, and had continued to block out her pain by becoming a workaholic:

> Finally, I burned out; my health broke . . . When I was given four days to live, I did a session with a friend and decided that I didn't want to die where Dad would have any chance of touching me. I felt so sick and vulnerable. I was dying. So I had my paramedic buddies smuggle me out of the hospital with portable oxygen and move me to a cabin high in the mountains.

> I lived alone there for six years; my only contact was with the abbot of the local monastery. He let me talk without judging me. He coached me to feel my anger and hurt. He taught me to fight fair, give up feeling sorry for myself, and how to affirm myself. He gave me books to read and insisted that I journal every minute I was conscious. I was too sick to leave my bed, but gradually, I began getting well.

Three months into phototherapy, Kay's vision improved to the point where she was able to use a seventeen-year-old pair of glasses for driving and could see clearly without glasses ten to twelve feet away. Her emotional health also improved dramatically — she no longer felt like an abandoned victim. Her sinus, bronchial, and asthmatic conditions disappeared, and x-rays of her lungs showed that they had totally healed. Since that time she has not had to visit her physician, has stopped taking all medications and injections, and, in her own words, is "healthy as a horse." Although treatment with the combination of red and yellow light initially brought up severe anxiety and fear as well as exacerbating many of Kay's physical symptoms, toward the completion of her treatment, viewing these same colors would elicit feelings of exhilaration and joy.

Kay is presently working full time as a therapist and college instructor of cognitive psychology. In a letter to me following her treatment, she concluded:

I came to work on my eyes. I left treatment having recovered *myself* and my eyesight. I've been able to process my old pain to the point where it almost feels like a story that happened to someone else. I no longer feel attached to the drama. I am no longer the helpless little kid. I survived it all! Now I'm learning to live my life one day at a time.

I have nearly completed my healing with my mother, and, last week, for the first time in my life, Dad was able to say, "I love you," with love in his eyes. I am so grateful I had the opportunities to hurt, to struggle, to grow strong in my ability to deal with tough situations and come out whole on the other side. Since I did it, anyone can. I have a depth of understanding and compassion now that no college course could ever teach me.

Now I won't have to say to my clients, "I don't know how you feel, because I've never been there." I have been there! I am now in the best possible position to support others in their healing. I am healing an impossible life. Now I know that everything is possible.

I am convinced that colored light therapy is destined to become "the drug of choice" in years to come! Light therapy releases the mental blocks that kids construct to maintain their balance in dysfunctional homes. The treatment is gentle; the results are profound.

Kay's healing is truly a miracle. It is clear that use of this light therapy within a safe environment provides an opportunity for individuals to feel, express, and release their fear, pain, anger, and so on, as these emotions surface, frequently resulting in a very deep *cellular transformation*. Old painful memories are lifted out of the body and mind, and thus the weed we call disease is pulled out by the roots. By increasing our awareness of our painful early experiences, which are the basis for the internal belief systems that chronically keep us out of balance, our bodies will automatically rebalance and heal themselves, as they are genetically programmed to do.

15

Light:
The Final
Frontier

Life is basically an energy experience. All of our human interactions, as well as our physiological functions, are vibrational in nature. The sun's vibrational energy is the most potent life-sustaining force in our very immediate "universe," which we call the *solar* system. It is now clear that different aspects, or frequencies, of this energy have different effects on our moods, behaviors, and vital functions. *Therefore, the biological receptivity of an organism to these different frequencies will determine which aspects of its functions and awareness will be stimulated and nourished.* Each separate frequency, or color of the spectrum, has *nutritional value,* and is the food for the initial development and constant evolvement of certain aspects of our being. Together, these frequencies unite into a rainbow of balanced nutrition that connects and synchronizes the vital functions of all organisms with the natural chronology of the cosmos.

It is my experience that our constantly changing states of consciousness determine the degree to which we are emotionally and biologically receptive. This, in turn, determines which portions of the spectrum we are attuned to (our vibrational experience) and, therefore, which ones we are more receptive to. Our total development is dependent upon the quality and specific aspects of universal light to which we are receptive. Light is that superterrestrial, natural force under which all life on Earth originates and develops.

BRINGING IN THE LIGHT

It is possible to change your own biological receptivity by bringing in the light. Imagine a transparent bar graph, as tall and wide as your body, with seven vertical columns of color, in the following order from left to right: red, orange, yellow, green, blue, indigo, and violet. Now imagine looking at yourself in a mirror. The transparent bar graph is on the surface of the mirror so that it is superimposed on the image of your body.

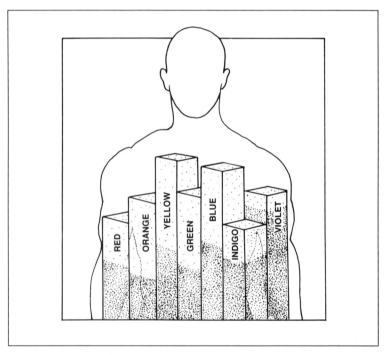

Figure 31. *Bar graph of color receptivity.*

Now close your eyes and visualize bringing in a beam of white light down through the top of your head, and notice that somewhere in your head the white light is prismatically broken into the seven colors of the rainbow so that each begins to fill up its respective column on the bar graph with a liquidlike paint. Wait for the columns to be filled to whatever degree they naturally fill, and then notice the level of each color in its column. Observe which of these nutritive color columns are filled and which ones seem to be lacking. How do you feel?

The colors that are low are like nutritional supplements that you are lacking and need. Visualize bringing each of these colors into your body one at a time, as if you are breathing them in through the top of your head, until each column is filled. How do you feel now?

Whenever you are feeling physically ill, emotionally upset, or just tired, consider taking yourself through this guided imagery. Notice what colors you are lacking, fill up your tanks, and you will probably find that you feel better. Do this at least once a day during stressful periods or just to occasionally check the levels at which you are assimilating light.

WHERE NO ONE HAS GONE BEFORE

This book has been about the journey to bring in the light. This journey began with the discoveries and intuitive knowledge of our pioneering ancestors, who, based on their writings, seemed to perform magic with light. Their wisdom laid the foundations for many of our modern scientific discoveries. The sun was once used as a general tonic to heal almost everything. Today, light and its component colors are being utilized in almost every aspect of science and medicine. Physicians, who once believed that only powerful, invasive drugs and technologies could have value in healing, are now beginning to appreciate the noninvasive power of light. Our other so-called "leading-edge technologies" in healing may soon be seen as "barbaric," as "Star Trek's" Dr. McCoy would say. Invasive medical approaches to treatment will become outdated as we enter the *light age*. Scalpels will be replaced by lasers, chemotherapy by phototherapy, prescription drugs by prescription colors, acupuncture needles by needles of light, eyeglasses by healthy eyes. Cancer will be a disease of the past; health and longevity will be the norm of the future.

The educational environment will change from windowless, colorless, and inappropriately illuminated classrooms to colorful, playful, stimulating classrooms with plenty of fresh air and sunlight. As a result, our children will be physically and emotionally healthier, more creative, and excited about learning.

Our working environments will become healing environments, as businesses and industries learn that happy, healthy people are more productive. Typical fluorescent lighting will be replaced by sun-simulating lamps. Sunshine will be recognized for its health-giving properties, and daily exposure will be recommended and scheduled into our work activities.

Our present psychotherapeutic approaches to emotional healing, such as traditional analysis, counseling, and medication, which are often designed to "make the pain go away," will be replaced. Instead, light therapy, designed to bring unresolved emotional issues to the surface, will be used to generate healthy expression and release of long-held pain, leading to self-respect, greater creativity, healthy relationships, and a new level of bodily health. The mind and body will no longer be looked upon as two separate entities. Our therapeutic techniques will treat the mind and body as one functioning whole system. This integration will propel humankind into greater feelings of wholeness, unity, and common purpose.

The 1990s are a time of accelerated awareness about all phases of human evolution. It is a critical period. Concerns over the environment, human and animal rights, health care, and world peace are forcing human beings to open their eyes, hearts, and minds further than ever before. It is time to stop raping the Earth and each other, and time to realize that we are all connected. Chopping down forests, killing animals, and treating the human body as a piece of equipment with replaceable parts are no longer acceptable actions. One hand must assist the other. The issues are bigger than any of us individually, yet by individually becoming living examples of what it means to be whole, healthy, caring, and loving beings, we each play a profoundly important role in the healing of our planet.

The *real* medicine of the future will recognize the connection between mind, body, and spirit, and treat them as one. Our technology will speak directly to the core of the body, so that its own wisdom can be the foundation for its healing. This new medicine will not treat disease — it will treat people. It will not focus only on the part — it will focus on the whole.

Rather than directing our eyes *outward*, looking for external causes to our internal imbalances, it is time to look *inward* at the parts of us that have been unreceptive to certain aspects of life, causing us to close down and become ill. The new medicine will not be invasive. It will challenge the body and mind, energetically, to reawaken. It will wake up those areas of ourselves that have been sleeping, and in so doing, it will impart the tools that our bodies need for healing.

The study of light affirms the interconnectedness of all things. It is a paradigm of the balance between the outside and the inside and is not much different from cellular physiology or, for that matter, human relationships. Dealing with an energy source that is both visible and nonvisible is also a reminder that both sides of life — what we can see and what we cannot see — are equally important to our development, growth, and evolution. That which is really going on in our lives can frequently be understood only by taking an illogical look.

Much pain and joy have been the substances washing the wounds of my life and clearing my eyes. We have entered an age when we must look at things from *nowhere* rather than experiencing them from only our own points of view and, thus, artificially coloring our realities. Years of personal experience have led me to this vision.

> The eyes were meant to see with.
> Give them a chance.
> Let them go.
> Let them see. Let yourself live.
> Let the light in!

APPENDIX A

Full-Spectrum Light Sources & Other Related Products

When the specifications for full-spectrum light sources were originally filed with the U.S. Food and Drug Administration, there were two primary factors that were considered. First was the color-rendering index (CRI), which is a rating of a bulb's ability to duplicate the near- and mid-bands of ultraviolet light and the entire visible spectrum of sunlight. A rating of 100 is an ideal source (the sun) and anything over 90 is considered full spectrum. The Vita-Lite, for example, has a CRI of 91, whereas a standard cool-white fluorescent light has a CRI of only 68. The second factor was Correlated Color Temperature, which measures the temperature at which a lamp burns. The original FDA specification was a range of 5,500 to 6,500 degrees Kelvin. Presently, a full-spectrum light source is any bulb that has a CRI of 90 or above and a color temperature between approximately 5,000 and 7,500 degrees Kelvin.

Duro-Test Corporation
9 Law Drive
Fairfield, NJ 07007
800-289-3876
Product: Vita-Lite

G.E. Lighting
Product Service
Nela Park
Cleveland, OH 44112
800-626-2000
Product: Chroma 50

North American Philips
200 Franklin Square Drive
Somerset, NJ 08873
Product: Colortone 50

GTE Products Corporation
U.S. Lighting Division
Danvers, MA 01923
800-225-5483
Product: Design 50

Ott Light Systems, Inc.
622 W. Arrellaga St., Suite D
Santa Barbara, CA 93101
800-234-3724 or 805-564-3467
Product: Ott Light

L.C.I. Lighting
24-hour order line: 800-999-4027
Product: Spectralite

Verilux Corporation
P.O. Box 7633
Vallejo, CA 94590
800-786-6850
Product: Complete Line

The Ott Light is an actual fixture that incorporates several innovations such as a separate UV bulb that allows the user to see when the UV has burned out, so it can be replaced (with normal full-spectrum tubes, it is impossible to tell when the UV portion has burned out); lead shielding on all cathodes to eliminate x-ray emissions; and a UV-transmitting diffuser with a special wire mesh that grounds radio-wave emissions.

LIGHTS FOR REVITALIZING FOOD AND WATER

Dr. Hazel R. Parcells
1605 Coal Ave., SE
Albuquerque, NM 87106
505-247-2744
Product: Thea-Lite

Kiva, Inc.
912 Broadway, NE
Albuquerque, NM 87102
505-242-5200
Product: Kiva Light

Thea-Lite combines light energy and a magnetic field to remove spray residues, metallics, pollutants, and additives from the food we eat every day, restoring the normal vitality of the food.

RECOMMENDATIONS FOR ANYONE UTILIZING FULL-SPECTRUM FLUORESCENT TUBES

1. Shield the cathodes (ends of the tubes) with lead impregnated tape (available through 3M Corp.) to eliminate x-ray emissions.

2. If possible, convert your system from AC to DC to eliminate the 60Hz flicker. If this is not possible, use an electronic ballast. This will increase the cycles from 60 to 25,000, thus reducing the flicker and saving energy.

3. Use UV-transmitting diffusers, egg-crate-type diffusers, or no diffuser at all. Standard diffusers absorb the UV portion of the spectrum.

APPENDIX B

College of Syntonic Optometry Practitioners

UNITED STATES

Arizona

Al Balthazor, O.D.
8003 E. Apache Trail
Mesa, AZ 85207
602-986-1601

Pamela S. Golden, Acupuncturist
3366 E. Evans
Phoenix, AZ 85032
602-971-1207

Arkansas

John D. Miller, O.D.
Box 926
Jacksonville, AR 72076
501-666-2020

Lyman Squires, O.D.
P.O. Box 424
Berryville, AR 72616
501-423-2576

California

Moses Albalas, O.D., Ph.D.
12732 W. Washington Blvd., Suite A
Los Angeles, CA 90066
213-306-3737

Curtis Baxstrom, O.D.
3636 N. Blackstone
Fresno, CA 93726
209-226-8161

Elliott Brainard, O.D., F.C.O.V.D.
2562 State St., Suite E
Carlsbad, CA 92008
619-434-5025

Dennis Chinn, O.D.
5151 N. Palm Ave., Suite 530
Fresno, CA 93704-2201
209-224-8302

Steven Cohn, O.D.
833 Dover Drive, Suite 9
Newport Beach, CA 92660
714-642-0292

Denise C. Davis, V.T., E.T., C.L.P.
1235 Summit Ave.
Cardiff, CA 92007
619-436-7632

John Downing, O.D., Ph.D.
100 Santa Rosa Plaza
Santa Rosa, CA 95401
707-526-1881

Dale A. Fast, O.D.
1111 Howe Ave., Suite 235
Sacramento, CA 95825
916-929-9162

Clifford A. Fukushima, O.D.
5501 Hillsdale Drive
Visalia, CA 93291
209-625-5464

C. William Harpur, O.D.
1288 Camino Del Rio N.
San Diego, CA 92108
619-692-1781

Lee Hartley, Ed.D.
4020 Moorpark Ave., Suite 117
San Jose, CA 95117
408-249-6943

Institute for Light Energy Research
449 Santa Fe Drive, Ste. 246
Encinitas, CA 92024
619-944-2934
800-326-8589

Larry A. Jebrock, O.D.
1702 Novato Blvd.
Novato, CA 94947
415-897-9691

Louis J. Katz, O.D., M.P.H., D.O.S.
4009 Governor Dr.
San Diego, CA 92122-3021
619-453-0444

Benjamin J. Kohn, O.D.
5051 Canyon Crest Dr., Suite 102
Riverside, CA 92507
714-686-3937

Bradford Murray, O.D.
1556 Carlson Way
San Jose, CA 95125
408-445-2020

Wayne Nishio, O.D.
1735 Minnewawa Ave., Suite 103
Clovis, CA 96312
209-299-3179

Samuel Pesner, O.D.
133 2nd St.
Los Altos, CA 94022
415-948-3700

Eldon Rosenow, O.D.
817 Coffee Rd., Bld. D
Modesto, CA 95355
209-524-9291

Marvin I. Schwartz, O.D., Ph.D.
3811 Florin Rd., Suite 9
Sacramento, CA 95823
916-421-3311/428-1133

Lawrence G. Simons, O.D.
9701 W. Pico Blvd., Suite 215
Los Angeles, CA 90035
310-284-8033

Philip B. Smith, O.D.
3636 4th Ave., Suite 200
San Diego, CA 92103
619-297-4331

Herb Solomon, O.D.
1180 South LaBrea
Los Angeles, CA 90035
213-933-9425

Gilbert Stocks, O.D.
321 W. Yosemite, Suite 300
Madera, CA 93637
209-674-0039

Daniel R. Taketa, O.D.
611 E. Ocean Ave.
Lompoc, CA 93436
805-736-7010

Daniel Ulseth, O.D.
200 Vera Ave.
Ripon, CA 95366
209-599-2216

Claude A. Valenti, O.D.
8950 Villa La Jolla Dr., Suite 1114
La Jolla, CA 92037
619-453-0442

Irving S. Werksman, O.D.
372 N. Moorpark Rd.
Thousand Oaks, CA 91360
(Metropolitan Los Angeles)
805-495-0446

Paul Yamashita, O.D.
1611 Lewis Street, Box 367
Kingsburg, CA 93631
209-897-2464

Shaw Yorizane, Jr., O.D.
5150 6th St., Suite 100
Fresno, CA 93710
209-222-6576

Colorado

Rebecca Hutchins, O.D., F.C.O.V.D.
3065 Center Green Dr., Suite 120
Boulder, CO 80301
303-443-7312

Jacob Liberman, O.D., Ph.D.
P.O. Box 4058
Aspen, CO 81612-4058
303-920-4413

John H. Philip, D.C.
75 S. 3rd Street
Carbondale, CO 81623
303-963-1575

M. Stuart Tessler, O.D., F.C.S.O.
6979 S. Holly Circle, Suite 105
Englewood, CO 80112
303-850-9499

Connecticut

Kenneth L. Burke, O.D.
175 Main St. South
Woodbury, CT 06798
203-263-3391
Fax 203-263-3390

Constantine J. Forkiotis, O.D.
437 Tunxis Hill Rd., Box 741
Fairfield, CT 06430
203-333-2772

Phyllis A. Liu, O.D.
570 Amiter Rd.
Woodbridge, CT 06525
203-624-5407

Florida

Melvin Apple, O.D.
900 NW 13th St.
Boca Raton, FL 33486
407-395-7074

Walter J. Chao, O.D.
7867 Pines Blvd.
Pembroke Pines, FL 33024
305-966-4335

William A. Clement, O.D.
P.O. Box 1099
123 W. Oak St.
Arcadia, FL 33821
813-494-2662

Philip Czyz, O.D.
21178 Olean Blvd., Unit A
Port Charlotte, FL 33952
813-629-1090

Mark B. Frank, D.C.
4900 Allen Rd.
Zephyr Hills, FL 33541
813-788-0496

Gayle H. Fuqua, O.D.
1635 South Ridgewood Ave.
South Daytona, FL 32119
904-760-7799

Kirby R. Hotchner, D.O.
3399 Ponce de Leon Blvd., Ste. 201
Coral Gables, FL 33134
305-529-1507

W.L. Howard, O.D.
Box 776
Wauchula, FL 33873
813-773-6459

Ralph F. Mead, O.D.
1225 E. Mt. Vernon
Orlando, FL 32803
407-896-4511

Albert A. Sutton, O.D.
820 Lakeview Dr.
Miami Beach, FL 33140
305-861-8415

Hanoch Talmor, M.D.
4400 NW 23rd Ave., Suite B
Gainesville, FL 32606
904-377-0015

John Walesby, O.D.
7110 Nebraska Ave.
Tampa, FL 33604
813-238-6471

Hawaii
Glen Swartwout, O.D.
P.O. Box 4991
Hilo, HI 96720
808-788-2442

Indiana
Pat McMillen, O.D.
319 Vigo Street
P.O. Box 138
Vincennes, IN 47591
812-882-0738

Iowa
Donald H. Hansen, O.D.
1923 Main St.
Davenport, IA 52803
319-324-3241

Kansas
Lowell Goodwin, O.D., F.C.O.V.D
704 N. Main St.
P.O. Box 638
Garden City, KS 67846
316-276-2261

L.L. McCormick, O.D.
1001 N. Main
Hutchinson, KS 67501
316-663-5417

Louis Mogel, O.D.
1001 N. Main
Hutchinson, KS 67501
316-663-5417

M.J. Philbrook, O.D.
7161 State Ave.
Kansas City, KS 66112
913-299-3548

Larry Young, O.D.
1001 N. Main
Hutchinson, KS 67501
316-663-5417

Maine
Bradford D. Smith, O.D.
15 Western Ave.
Augusta, ME 04330
207-623-2020

Maryland
Sanford R. Cohen, O.D.
3933 Ferrara Dr.
Silver Spring, MD 20906
301-946-2550

Massachusetts
Nancy Berkan, M.Ed., (Ph.D., 1995)
Ellery St.
Cambridge, MA 02138
617-661-5955

Isabelle B. King, Ph.D.
70 Run Hill Rd.
Brewster, MA 02631
508-896-3858

Earl H. Lizotte, O.D.
P.O. Box 711
176 Main St.
East Hampton, MA 01027
413-527-4881

Solomon K. Slobins, O.D.
1200 Robeson St.
Fall River, MA 02720
508-673-1251

Cathy Stern, O.D.
27 Harvard St.
Brookline, MA 02146
617-277-7754

Minnesota
Patrick J. Flanagan, O.D.
4473 Lake Elmo Ave. N.
Lake Elmo, MN 55042
612-779-6780

Robert E. Zwicky, O.D.
2550 Univ. Ave. W., Suite 163 S.
St. Paul, MN 55114
612-645-8124

Missouri
David J. Luke, O.D.
121 N. Allen
P.O. Box 82
Centralia, MO 65240
314-581-3848

Nebraska
R.A. Manthey, O.D.
237 S. 70th St.
Esquire Plaza, Suite 101
Lincoln, NE 68510
402-483-0042

New Hampshire
Shirley S. Snow, N.D., D.N.B.
755 Straw Hill
Manchester, NH 03104
603-644-4525

New Jersey
Herman Cohn, O.D.
217 Glenridge Ave.
Montclair, NJ 07042

Rudolf S. Domino, O.D.
228 Plainfield Ave.
Edison, NJ 08817
201-985-5009

Jay Feder, O.D.
17 Icemeadow
Matawan, NJ 07747
201-583-9192

Irving Grossman, O.D.
525 Belford Rd.
Cranbury, NJ 08512
201-655-1531

David E. Kraus, O.D.
9226 Kennedy Blvd.
North Bergen, NJ 07047
201-861-7202

Stanley H. Levine, O.D.
240 Amboy Ave.
Metuchen, NJ 08840
201-548-3636

Stephen R. Niemiera, O.D.
474 Amboy Ave.
Perth Amboy, NJ 08861
908-826-9330

Andrew Pritchard, O.D.
702 Stillholse Land
Marlton, NJ 08053
609-596-9126

Bruce Rosenfeld, O.D.
112 W. Franklin Ave., D-7
Pennington, NJ 08534
609-737-7147

Russell Sinoway, O.D.
309 S. Orange Ave.
So. Orange, NJ 07079
201-763-3511

Charles Sosis, O.D.
Oak Ridge Pkwy & Cardinal Dr.
Box 383
Toms River, NJ 08754
201-240-0020

Raymond P. Taub, O.D.
1 W. Cliff St.
Somerville, NJ 08876
201-725-2915

A. Van Beveren, Ph.D.
952 Rt. 518
Skillman, NJ 08558
609-924-7337

Vincent R. Vicci, Jr., O.D.
P.O. Box 904
123 N. Union Ave.
Cranford, NJ 07016
908-272-1133

James Washington, O.D.
104 S. Munn Ave.
East Orange, NJ 07018
201-675-5392

Harold Wiener, O.D.
Marc Wiener, O.D.
64 Ridge Rd.
North Arlington, NJ 07032
201-991-2211

New Mexico
Robert B. Pomeranz, O.D.
651 Campfire Rd. SE
Rio Rancho, NM 87124
505-892-1437

Sam Berne, O.D.
1300 Luisa St., Suite 4
Santa Fe, NM 87505
505-984-2030

New York
Jay M. Cohen, O.D.
55 W. 11th St.
New York, NY 10011
212-989-4238

Marc Grossman, O.D.
20 Chestnut St.
Rye, NY 10580
914-967-1740
3 Paradise Lane
New Paltz, NY 12561
914-255-3228

Joseph Shapiro, O.D.
80 Fifth Ave., Suite 1105
New York, NY 10011
212-255-2240

Larry B. Wallace, O.D.
322 N. Aurora St.
Ithaca, NY 14850
607-277-4749

Gerald Wintrob, O.D.
380 Marlborough Rd.
Brooklyn, NY 11226
718-856-2020

North Carolina
James C. Herring, O.D.
2409 N. Elm St.
Lumberton, NC 28358
910-739-8141

Ohio
Paul Newman, O.D.
279 S. Main St.
Akron, OH 44308
216-253-1627

Oklahoma
Carl Mahaney, O.D.
908 N. Callie Ave.
Tahlequah, OK 74464
918-456-3504

Oregon

Larry K. Burr, O.D.
1631 Oak St.
Eugene, OR 97401
503-342-4243

Sandra K. Landis, O.D.
14385 SW Allen Blvd., Suite 102
Beaverton, OR 97005
503-646-8592

Pennsylvania

Sam Berne, O.D.
313 N. Newtown St. Rd.
P.O. Box 107
Newtown Square, PA 19073
215-356-1889

Stuart M. Clark, O.D.
115 Main St.
Trappe, PA 19426
610-489-0870

Ellis S. Edelman, O.D.
313 N. Newtown St. Rd.
P.O. Box 107
Newtown Square, PA 19073
610-356-1889

Steven J. Gallop, O.D.
313 N. Newtown St. Rd.
P.O. Box 107
Newtown Square, PA 19073
610-356-7425

Betsy J. Hancock, O.D.
21 E. 5th St.
Bloomsburg, PA 17815
717-784-2131

Leonard B. Krachman, O.D.
403 Ave. of the States
Chester, PA 19013
610-874-9404

Jacob Parker, O.D., Ph.D.
8595 Bustleton Ave.
Philadelphia, PA 19152
215-722-1133

Bruce Rosenfeld, O.D.
4817 Kings Rd.
Doylestown, PA 18901
215-348-5130

Christa Roser, O.D.
714 N. 5th St.
Reading, PA 19601
215-375-8526

Puerto Rico

Ana Maria Pico, O.D.
Calle 2 #J-12A, Ext. Hnas Dávila
Bayamón, P.R. 00619
809-780-0677

Wanda M. Tort, O.D.
Calle 2 #J-12A, Ext. Hnas Dávila
Bayamón, P.R. 00619
809-780-0677

Rhode Island

Edward I. Lyons, O.D.
989 Reservoir Ave.
Cranston, RI 02910
401-943-1122

Dr. George S. Shola
180A Danielson Pke.
P.O. Box 243
N. Scituate, RI 02857
401-647-3106

South Carolina

Timothy D. Brewerton, M.D.
Medical University of South Carolina
Dept. of Psychiatry
171 Ashley Ave.
Charleston, SC 29425
803-792-7183
Fax 803-792-0257

John Brinkley, O.D.
426 Bush River Rd.
Columbia, SC 29210
803-798-8111

Alva Pack, O.D.
399 E. Henry St.
Spartanburg, SC 29302
803-585-0208
Fax 803-573-7132

South Dakota
Charles Howlin, O.D.
3712 S. Western
Sioux Falls, SD 57101
605-332-2231

Texas
Dhavid Cooper, O.D.
(Researcher)
2055 Westheimer, #115
Houston, TX 77098
713-520-6600

David Saul Mora, O.D., Ph.D.
1601 Corpus Cristi
Laredo, TX 78043
512-726-1007/726-9001

Teresa Peck, O.D.
1713 E. Hwy 35
Angleton, TX 77515
409-849-7321

A.C. Pruneda, Jr., O.D.
700 Zarzamora, Suite 201
San Antonio, TX 78207
512-436-8808

Ted Vorster, O.D., M.S.
3729 Westheimer
Houston, TX 77027
713-993-0344

U.S. Virgin Islands
Donald E. Young, O.D.
Upper Havensight Mall
P.O. Box 7939
St. Thomas, U.S. Virgin Islands 00801
809-774-6315

Virginia
Dennis R. Cantwell, O.D.
7611 Little River Tpk., #303
Annandale, VA 22003
703-941-3937

Craig S. Dacales, O.D.
4001 Fair Ridge Dr., Ste. 305
Fairfax, VA 22033
703-385-6134

Washington
George N. Dever, O.D.
1511 3rd Ave., Suite 411
Seattle, WA 98101
206-624-0737

John Ellson, O.D.
Box 589
Pasco, WA 99301
509-547-6366

Sidney Hays, O.D.
7902 W. 27th St.
Tacoma, WA 98466
206-564-9262

Carl Olson, O.D.
18534 29th NE
Seattle, WA 98155
206-782-6071

Wisconsin
Robert B. Bower, O.D.
2301 - 75th St.
Kenosha, WI 53140
414-654-6005

AUSTRALIA

Peter Fairbanks
45 Lydiard St. South
Ballarat, Victoria
Australia 3350
053 323 421
Fax 053 317 336

Simon Grbevski, O.D.
458 Princes Hwy., 1st Floor
Rockdale, Australia 2216
597-3030
Fax 61-2-597-6413

BELGIUM

Bernard Cassiers, O.D.
Lange Leemstraat 142
2018 Antwerpen, Belgium
03-230-9799
Rooigemlaan, 99
9000 Gent
09-226-04-24

NETHERLANDS

Jan W. Dijkhof, O.D.
Dijk 46
1811 MC. Alkmaar
Netherlands
072-117235

CANADA

Alberta

Sonja G. Hagemann, O.D.
4820 Northland Dr., NW
Calgary, Alberta
Canada T3B 4N9
403-286-5135

British Columbia

James C. Thompson, O.D.
3-3260 Edgemont Blvd.
N. Vancouver, B.C.
Canada V7R 2P2
604-987-4224

Manitoba

Doug Holroyd, O.D.
39 Royal Road N.
Portage, La Prairie, Manitoba
Canada RIN 1W8
204-857-8559

Gerard G. Murray, O.D.
39 Royal Road N.
Portage, La Prairie, Manitoba
Canada RIN 1W8
204-857-4760

Ontario

June G. Robertson, O.D.
1515 Rebecca St., Suite 208
Hopedale Mall
Oakville, Ontario
Canada L6L 5G8
416-827-4711

Howard C. Thompson, O.D.
4 Algonquin Blvd.
Bramalea, Ontario
Canada L6T 1R8
416-793-2020

Rick H. Thompson, O.D.
4 Algonquin Blvd.
Bramalea, Ontario
Canada L6T 1R8
416-793-2020

APPENDIX C

Wohlfarth's Colors for Walls

Dr. Wohlfarth used the following colors in his school studies:

1. Warm light yellow (Glidden 73-85) on the three walls the students were facing

2. Warm light blue (Glidden 77-30) on the rear wall and the vertical surfaces of the student desks facing the teachers

3. Blue (Glidden 77-81) for the "blackboards"

4. Warm light yellow to stimulate the slow students, and warm light blue to relax hyperkinetic students in special-education classrooms

5. Warm golden-gray (Glidden 78-69) for the carpets

Glidden Company products were used because of their widespread availability in the United States and Canada.

Glidden Company
900 Union Commerce Bldg.
Cleveland, OH 44115
216-344-8000

These colors are copyrighted and can be used only with permission from Prof. Dr. Harry Wohlfarth, Colorpsychodynamic Design, Ltd., 1101, 11025-82nd Ave., Edmonton, Alberta, Canada T6G 0T1.

APPENDIX D

Clinical Investigators Utilizing Phototherapy
and Photofrin in the Treatment of Cancer

Dr. Oscar J. Balchum
St. Francis Medical Center
3630 E. Imperial Hwy., Room 253
Lynwood, CA 90262
213-226-7906

Dr. George Fisher
Clinical Professor of Medicine
University of Southern California
Goleta Valley Community Hospital
601 East Arrellaga St., #101
Santa Barbara, CA 93103
805-963-2029

Dr. Warren Grundfest
Cedars-Sinai Medical Center
8700 Beverly Blvd., Room 8215
Los Angeles, CA 90048
213-855-4685

Dr. Stephen Heier
Director, Edoscopy Unit
New York Medical College
Westchester County Medical Center
Dept. of Gastroenterology
Valhalla, NY 10595
914-285-7337

Dr. Steven Lam
Vancouver General Hospital
Dept. of Medicine
#102 - 2775 Heather St.
Vancouver, B.C. V5Z 3J5
604-875-4122

Dr. Norman Marcon
Chief, Div. of Gastroenterology
Wellesley Hospital
#121 Elsie K. Jones Bldg.
160 Wellesley St. East
Toronto, Ontario M4Y 1J3
416-926-7039

Dr. James McCaughan
Grant Laser Center
Laser Medical Research Foundation
323 East Towne St.
Columbus, OH 43215
614-221-2643

Dr. Unyime Nseyo
VA Medical Center
150 Muir Rd.
Martinez, CA 94553
415-228-6800

Dr. Anne-Marie Regal
Roswell Park Memorial Inst.
666 Elm St.
Buffalo, NY 14263
716-845-8577

Dr. Bryan Shumaker
North Woodward Urologic Assoc.
909 Woodward Ave.
Pontiac, MI 48053
313-338-4038

APPENDIX E

Partial Directory of Practitioners Working with SAD

For general information about light treatments, national and international referrals to research volunteer programs, and a listing of manufacturers and suppliers, contact:

Society for Light Treatment
and Biological Rhythms (SLTBR)
P.O. Box 478
Wilsonville, OR 97070
503-694-2404

UNITED STATES

Arkansas

Frederick Guggenheim, M.D.
Chairman, Dept. of Psychiatry
University of Arkansas for Medical
  Sciences
4301 W. Markham, Slot 589
Little Rock, AR 72205
501-661-5483

California

Daniel F. Kripke, M.D.
Scripps Clinic
10666 N. Torrey Pines Rd.
La Jolla, CA 92037
619-554-8087

Barbara L. Parry, M.D.
Department of Psychiatry, T-004
UCSD, 225 Dickinson St.
San Diego, CA 92103
619-543-5592

Hugh Ridlehuber, M.D.
215 N. San Mateo Dr.
San Mateo, CA 94401
415-579-5785

Colorado

Marvin Robbins, M.D.
4770 Iliff Ave.
Denver, CO 80222
303-756-1308

Connecticut

Edward W. Allen, M.D.
504 Goose Lane
Guilford, CT 06437
203-453-5554

Francine C. Howland, M.D.
45 Trumbull St.
New Haven, CT 06510
203-624-3516

Lawrence N. Rossi, M.D.
Institute of Living
200 Retreat Ave.
Hartford, CT 06106
203-241-6889

Seasonal Affective Disorders Team
L&M Hospital Counseling Services
365 Montauk Ave.
New London, CT 06320
203-444-5125

District of Columbia Metropolitan Area

Norman E. Rosenthal, M.D.
Thomas A. Wehr, M.D.
Seasonal Studies Program
National Institute of Mental Health
Building 10, Room 4S-239
9000 Rockville Pike
Bethesda, MD 20892
301-496-2141 or 496-0500

Florida

Robert G. Skwerer, M.D.
Sarasota Palms Hospital
1650 S. Osprey Ave.
Sarasota, FL 34239
813-366-6070

Idaho

Winslow R. Hunt, M.D.
155 2nd Ave.
Pocatello, ID 83201
208-232-3423

Illinois

Henry W. Lahmeyer, M.D.
Department of Psychiatry
University of Illinois, Box 6998
M/C 913912 S. Wood St.
Chicago, IL 60612
312-996-9518

Indiana

Richard H. Spector, M.D.
9250 Columbia Ave.
Munster, IN 46321
219-836-0810

Boghos Yerevanian, M.D.
Kingwood Hospital
3714 S. Franklin St.
Michigan City, IN 46360
219-873-1610

Iowa

Bill Yates, M.D.
Keith L. Rogers, M.D.
Department of Psychiatry
University of Iowa
500 Newton Rd.
Iowa City, IA 52242
319-353-6218

Kentucky

Edward Goldenberg, M.D.
Behavioral Medicine Group
1401 Harrodsburg Rd., Suite A-420
Lexington, KY 40504
606-278-0317

Maryland

Seasonal Studies Program
National Institute of Mental Health
(see listing under District of Columbia Metropolitan Area)

Massachusetts

Gary S. Sachs, M.D.
Massachusetts General Hospital
15 Parkman St., ACC-715
Boston, MA 02114
617-726-3488

Martin H. Teischer, M.D.
McLean Hospital
115 Mill St.
Belmont, MA 02178
617-855-2970

Missouri

Dale J. Anderson, M.D.
14377 Woodlake Dr., Suite #301
St. Louis, MO 63017
314-576-6493

Nebraska
Robert G. Osborne, M.D.
2221 S. 17th St., Suite 110
Lincoln, NE 68502
402-476-7557

Kay M. Shilling, M.D.
7602 Pacific St., Suite 302
Omaha, NE 68114
402-393-4355

New Hampshire
John P. Docherty, M.D.
Brookside Hospital
11 Northwest Blvd.
Nashua, NH 03603
603-886-5000

John W. Raasoch, M.D.
331 Main St.
Keene, NH 03431
603-357-4400

New Jersey
Jeffrey T. Apter, M.D.
Princeton Psychiatric Centers
330 N. Harrison St., #6
Princeton, NJ 08540
609-921-3555

Robert E. McGrath, Ph.D.
Department of Psychology
Fairleigh Dickinson University
Teaneck, NJ 07666
201-692-2300

New York
Joseph Deltito, M.D.
21 Bloomingdale Rd.
Cornell University Medical Center
White Plains, NY 10605
914-997-5967

James W. Flax, M.D.
2420 N. Main St.
New City, NY 10956
914-638-3358

Richard Kavey, M.D.
725 Irving Ave., Suite 409
Syracuse, NY 13210
315-470-7367

NY/NJ/CT-Area Research Volunteers
(free treatment):
Michael Terman, Ph.D.
Light Therapy Unit
New York Psychiatric Institute
722 W. 168th St., Box 50
New York, NY 10032
212-960-5714

NY/NJ/CT-Area Clinical Service for
Private Patients:
Light Therapy Center, Dept. of
Behavioral Medicine
The Presbyterian Hospital
(Manhattan)
212-960-2200, ext. 697

Leslie L. Powers, M.D.
15 W. 75th St.
New York, NY 10023
212-724-5222

Ohio
Steven Dilsaver, M.D.
Dept. of Psychiatry
Div. of Psychopharmacology
Ohio State University
473 W. 12th St.
Columbus, OH 43210-1228
614-293-5254

Gregory G. Young, M.D.
1735 Big Hill Rd.
Dayton, OH 45439
513-293-2507

Oregon
George C. D. Kjaer, M.D.
132 E. Broadway, Suite 301
Eugene, OR 97401
503-686-2027

Pennsylvania

Karl Doghramji, M.D.
Sleep Disorders Center
Dept. of Psychiatry and Human
    Behavior
Jefferson Medical College
1015 Walnut St.
Philadelphia, PA 19107
215-928-5045

David E. Thomas, M.D.
211 N. Whitfield St., #800
Pittsburgh, PA 15206
412-363-7368

South Carolina

Timothy D. Brewerton, M.D.
Medical University of South Carolina
Department of Psychiatry and
    Behavioral Sciences
171 Ashley Ave.
Charleston, SC 29425-0742
803-792-4795

Texas

John Cain, M.D.
Department of Psychiatry
University of Texas at Dallas
5323 Harry Hines Blvd.
Dallas, TX 75230
214-688-3300

Vermont

Ray C. Abney, M.D.
75 Linden St.
Brattleboro, VT 05301
802-257-7785, ext. 218

Edward Mueller, M.D.
Department of Mental Health
    Services, Inc.
78 S. Main St., Box 222
Rutland, VT 05701
802-775-2381/775-2386

Virginia

Bruce E. Baker, M.D.
150 Olde Greenwich Drive, Suite J
Fredericksburg, VA 22401
703-898-5533

Seasonal Studies Program
National Institute of Mental Health
(see listing under District of Colum-
    bia Metropolitan Area)

Washington

David H. Avery, M.D.
Harborview Medical Center, ZA-99
325 9th Ave.
Seattle, WA 98104
206-223-3425

Carla Hellekson, M.D.
Providence Sleep Disorders Center
500 17th Ave.
P.O. Box C-34008
Seattle, WA 98124
206-326-5366

Wisconsin

Nancy E. Barklage, M.D.
Center for Affective Disorders
Department of Psychiatry
University of Wisconsin Hospital and
    Clinics
600 Highland Dr.
Madison, WI 53792
608-263-6087

Steven V. Hansen, M.D.
1220 Dewey Ave.
Milwaukee, WI 53213
414-258-2600

CANADA

Quebec

Hami Iskandar, M.D.
Douglas Hospital Research Center
6875 Lasalle Blvd.
Verdun, Quebec H4H 1R3
514-761-6131

N.P. Vasavan Nair, M.D.
Douglas Hospital Research Center
6875 Lasalle Blvd.
Verdun, Quebec H4H 1R3
514-761-6131, ext. 23330

NOTES

CHAPTER 1

1. D. Bohm, "Of Matter and Meaning: The Super-Implicate Order," *ReVision* (Spring, 1983).

2. E. Keister, Jr., "Living Without Light," *Science Illustrated* 2, no. 7 (Mar./Apr. 1989): pp. 26-32.

3. L. Clark, *Ancient Art of Color Therapy* (New York: Pocket Books, 1975).

4. Z. Kime, *Sunlight* (Penryn, CA: World Health Publications, 1980).

5. Ibid.

6. A. Szent-Gyorgyi, *Introduction to a Submolecular Biology* (New York: Academic Press, 1960).

7. A. Szent-Gyorgyi, *Bioelectronics* (New York: Academic Press, 1968).

8. K. Martinek and I.V. Berezin, "Artificial Light-Sensitive Enzymatic Systems as Chemical Amplifiers of Weak Light Signals," *Photochemistry and Photobiology* 29 (Mar. 1979): pp. 637-650.

9. Z. Kime, *Sunlight* (Penryn, CA: World Health Publications, 1980).

CHAPTER 2

1. P. Webbink, *The Power of the Eyes* (New York: Springer).

2. A. Wimmer, "Der Einfluss der Erblindung in der Kindheit auf die Entwicklung des Körpers, auf das Gemüt und den Geist," *Jahresber-Königl-Blindenanstalt* (München, 1856).

3. B. Jensen, *The Science and Practice of Iridology* (Escondido, CA: Bernard Jensen, D.C., 1974).

4. R.B. Morgan, "Nutrition, Stress and the Visual Pathway" (Lecture presented at 2d annual South Eastern Conf., Atlanta, 1981).

5. P. Buffington, "The Psychology of Eyes," *Sky* (Feb. 1984): pp. 92-96.

6. R. Bandler and J. Grinder, *Frogs Into Princes* (Moab, UT: Real People Press, 1979).

7. B. Jensen, *The Science and Practice of Iridology* (Escondido, CA: Bernard Jensen, D.C., 1974).

8. F. Hollwich, *Ophthalmology* (Stuttgart-New York: Georg Thieme Verlag, 1979).

9. B. Jensen, *The Science and Practice of Iridology* (Escondido, CA: Bernard Jensen, D.C., 1974).

10. F. Hollwich, *The Influence of Ocular Light Perception on Metabolism in Man and in Animal* (New York: Springer-Verlag, 1979).

11. R. Greving, "Beitrage zur Anatomie des Zwischenhirns and seiner Funktion, der anatomische Verlauf eines Faserbundels des N. opticus beim Menschen (Tr. supraopticothalamicus), zugleich ein Beitrag zur Anatomie des unteren Thalamusstiels," *Graefes Arch.* 115 (1925): p. 523.

12. E. Frey, "Mitteilung uber die Existenz eines hypothalamisch-optischen Bundels. Sitzungsber. II" (Internat. Neurol. Kongr., London 1935), *Rev. Neurol.*(1935), p. 2.

13. E. Frey, "Uber die hypothalamische Optikuswurzel des Hundes," *Bull. d. Schweiz. Akad. Med. Wiss.* 7 (1951): p. 115.

14. E. Frey, "Neue anatomische Ergebnisse zur Phylogenie der Sehfunktion," *Beih. Klin. Mbl. Augenheilk.* (1955): p. 23.

15. H. Becher, "Uber ein vegetatives Kerngebiet and neurosekretorische Leistungen der Ganglienzellen der Netzhaut," *Klin. Mbl. Augenheilk. Beih.* 23 (1955): p. 1.

16. H. Knoche, "Die Vergindung der Retina mit den vegetativen Zentren des Zwischenhirns und der Hypophyse," *Verh. Anat. Ges. Stockholm* 103 (1956): p. 140.

17. S. Blumcke, "Zur Frage einer Nervenfaserverbindung zwischen Retina und Hypothalamus," *Z. Zellforsch.* 48 (1958): p. 261.

18. A.E. Hendrickson, N. Wagoner, and W.M. Cowan, "An Autoradiographic and Electron Microscopic Study of Retino-Hypothalamic Connections," *Z. Zellforsch.*, 135 (1972): p. 1.

19. R.Y. Moore, "Retinohypothalamic Projection in Mammals: A Comparative Study," *Brain Research* 49 (1973): p. 403.

20. H.G. Hartwig, "Electron Microscopic Evidence for a Retinohypothalamic Projection to the Suprachiasmatic Nucleus of *Passer Domesticus*," *Cell Tissue Research* 153 (1974): p. 89.

21. J. Lopiparo, "Phototherapy: Will Color Be the Next Medical Frontier?" *OP/The Osteopathic Physician* (July 1978): pp. 36-39.

22. E.W. Bovard, "A Concept of Hypothalamic Functioning," *Perspective on Biological Medicine* 5: pp. 52-60.

23. S. Fulder, *The Tao of Medicine* (New York: Destiny Books, 1982).

CHAPTER 3

1. B. Fellman, "A Clockwork Gland," *Science* (May 1985): pp. 76-83.

2. J.A. Kappers, "A Survey of Advances in Pineal Research," in *The Pineal Gland*, vol. 1, ed. R.J. Reiter (Boca Raton, FL: CRC Press, 1981): pp. 1-25.

3. S.S. Erlich and J.L.J. Apuzzo, "The Pineal Gland: Anatomy, Physiology, and Clinical Significance," *Journal of Neurosurgery* (1985): pp. 321-341.

4. R.J. Reiter, "The Pineal Gland: An Important Link to the Environment," *NIPS* 1 (Dec. 1986): pp. 202-205.

5. D. Benningfield, "Spring Forward," *Spirit* (January 1990).

6. B. Rensberger, "Biological Clock Clue in Brain," *The Washington Post*, Oct. 17, 1988.

7. D.C. Klein, "Direct Tie Discovered Between Pineal, Brain," *Brain/Mind Bulletin* 11, no. 8 (Apr. 1986): p. 1.

8. I. McIntyre, "Small Amount of Light Shown Capable of Diminishing Body's Melatonin Level," *Brain/Mind Bulletin* 15, no. 4 (Jan. 1990): pg. 7.

9. L. Lohmeier, "Let the Sun Shine In," *East West*, July 1986, pp. 36-39.

10. F. Hollwich, *The Influence of Ocular Light Perception on Metabolism in Man and in Animal* (New York: Springer-Verlag, 1979).

11. F. Hollwich and B. Dieckhues, "Endocrine System and Blindness," *German Medical Monthly* 1 (1971c): p. 22.

12. R. Relkin, "Miscellaneous Effects of the Pineal," in *The Pineal Gland*, ed. R. Relkin (New York: Elsevier Biomed, 1983): pp. 247-272.

13. H. Samis et al, "Aging and Temporal Organization," in *Interventions in Aging*, ed. R. Walker and R. Cooper (New York: Marcel Dekker, Inc., 1983): pp. 397-419.

14. W. Pierpaoli, "Melatonin Extends Rat Lives," *Brain/Mind Bulletin* 13, no. 9 (June 1988): pp. 1, 8.

15. Author Unknown, "The Pineal Gland and Aging," *Complementary Medicine* (Nov./Dec. 1986): pp. 47-51.

CHAPTER 4

1. C. Eastlake and J. Murray, trans., *Goethe's Theory of Colors* (London: 1840).

2. R. Steiner, *Colour* (London: Rudolf Steiner Press, 1982).

3. F. Birren, *Color Psychology and Color Healing* (Secaucus, NJ: The Citadel Press, 1961).

4. M. Lüscher, *The Lüscher Color Test* (New York: Washington Square Press, 1969).

5. R.M. Hill and E. Marg, "Single-cell Responses of the Nucleus of the Transpeduncular Tract in Rabbit to Monochromatic Light on the Retina," *Journal of Neurophysiology* 26 (1963): p. 249.

6. S.V. Krakov, "Color Vision and Autonomic Nervous System," *Journal of the Optical Society of America* (June 1942).

7. R.M. Gerard, "Differential Effects of Colored Lights on Psychophysiological Functions" (Ph.D. diss., University of California at Los Angeles, 1958).

8. H. Wohlfarth, "Psychological Evaluation of Experiments to Assert the Effects of Color-Stimuli Upon the Autonomic Nervous System," *Exerpta Medica, Neurology and Psychiatry* 2, no. 4 (1958).

9. B.S. Aaronson, "Color Perception and Affect," *American Journal of Clinical Hypnosis* 14 (1971): pp. 38-42.

10. J.J. Plack and J. Schick, "The Effects of Color on Human Behavior," *Journal of the Association for Study in Perception* 9 (1974): pp. 4-16.

11. G. Trexler, *The World of Light, Color, Health and Behavior* (Fairfield, IA: Self-Published, 1985).

12. R. Hodr, "Phototherapy of Hyperbilirubinemia in Premature Infants," translated from *Ceskoslovenska' Pediatrie* 26 (Feb. 1971): pp. 80-82.

13. R.J. Cremer, P.W. Perrman and D.H. Richards, "Influence of Light on Hyperbilirubinemia in Infants," *Lancet* 1 (1958): p. 1094.

14. J.R. Lucey, "Neonatal Jaundice and Phototherapy," *Pediatric Clinics of North America* 19, no. 4 (1972): pp. 1-7.

15. R. Hodr, "Phototherapy of Hyperbilirubinemia in Premature Infants," translated from *Ceskoslovenska' Pediatrie* 26 (Feb. 1971): pp. 80-82.

16. C. Houck, "The Case Against Artificial Light," *New York*, Dec. 4, 1978.

17. S.F. McDonald, "Effect of Visible Light Waves on Arthritis Pain: A Controlled Study," *International Journal of Biosocial Research* 3, no. 2 (1982): pp. 49-54.

18. J. Anderson, *Brain/Mind Bulletin* 15, no. 4 (Jan. 1990): p. 1.

19. A.G. Schauss, "Tranquilizing Effect of Color Reduces Aggressive Behavior and Potential Violence," *The Journal of Orthomolecular Psychiatry* 8, no. 4 (1979): pp. 218-221.

20. R.J. Pellegrini, A.G. Schauss, and T.J. Birk, "Leg Strength as a Function of Exposure to Visual Stimuli of Different Hues," *Bulletin of The Psychonomic Society* 16, no. 2 (1980): pp. 111-112.

21. L. Gruson, "Color Has Powerful Effect on Behavior, Researchers Assert," *The New York Times*, Oct. 19, 1982.

22. K. Costigan, "How Color Goes to Your Head," *Science Digest*, Dec. 1984.

23. A.G. Schauss, "The Physiological Effect of Color on the Suppression of Human Aggression: Research on Baker-Miller Pink," *International Journal of Biosocial Research* 72 (1985): pp. 55-64.

24. G. Legwold, "Color-Boosted Energy: How Lights Affect Muscle Action," *American Health*, May 1988.

25. J.N. Ott, "Color and Light: Their Effects on Plants, Animals, and People," *Journal of Biosocial Research* 7, part I (1985).

26. A. Fisher, "Light: Nature's Mysterious Essential Gift," *Geo Magazine* 3, Oct. 1981, pp. 66-78.

CHAPTER 5

1. D.B. Harmon, "The Coordinated Classroom." (Grand Rapids, MI: American Seating Company, 1951).

2. J.N. Ott, *Exploring the Spectrum* (a film by John Ott).

3. J.N. Ott, "Color and Light: Their Effects on Plants, Animals, and People," *Journal of Biosocial Research* 7, part I (1985).

4. I.M. Sharon, R.P. Feller, and S.W. Burney, "The Effects of Lights of Different Spectra on Caries Incidence in the Golden Hamster," *Archives of Oral Biology* 16, no. 12 (1971): pp. 1427-1431.

5. E.C. McBeath and T.F. Zuker, "The Role of Vitamin D in the Control of Dental Caries in Children," *Journal of Nutrition* 15 (1938): p. 547.

6. B.R. East, "Mean Annual Hours of Sunshine and Incidence of Dental Caries," *American Journal of Public Health* 29 (1939): p. 777.

7. L. Hays, "Which Came First, Low Cholesterol Egg or Happier Chicken," *The Wall Street Journal* 210, no. 113, Dec. 8, 1987.

8. J.N. Ott, "Color and Light: Their Effects on Plants, Animals, and People," *Journal of Biosocial Research* 7, part I (1985).

9. R. Altschul and I.H. Herman, "Ultraviolet Irradiation and Cholesterol Metabolism, Seventh Annual Meeting of the American Society for the Study of Arteriosclerosis," *Circulation* 8 (1953): p. 438.

10. Z. Kime, *Sunlight* (Penryn, CA: World Health Publications, 1980).

11. F. Hollwich and B. Dieckhues, "The Effect of Natural and Artificial Light Via the Eye on the Hormonal and Metabolic Balance of Animal and Man," *Ophthalmologica* 180, no. 4 (1980): pp. 188-197.

12. Dorothy A. Bernoff, personal correspondence with author, Nov. 11, 1989.

13. Personal conversations with Orie Bachechi from 1986-1990.

CHAPTER 6

1. F. Birren, *Color Psychology and Color Healing* (Secaucus, NJ: Citadel Press, 1961).

2. A. Fisher, "Light: Nature's Mysterious Essential Gift," *Geo Magazine 3*, Oct. 1981, pp. 66-78.

3. A.J. Pleasanton, *Blue and Sun-Lights* (Philadelphia: Claxton, Remsen and Haffelfinger, 1876).

4. S. Pancoast, *Blue and Red Lights* (Philadelphia: J.M. Stoddart and Co., 1877).

5. E.D. Babbitt, *The Principles of Light and Color* (East Orange, NJ: Self-Published, 1896).

6. Z. Kime, *Sunlight* (Penryn, CA: World Health Publications, 1980).

7. Ibid.

8. L. Lohmeier, "Let the Sun Shine In," *East West*, July 1986, p. 39.

9. Z. Kime, *Sunlight* (Penryn, CA: World Health Publications, 1980).

10. D.P. Ghadiali, *Spectro-Chrome Metry Encyclopedia* (Malaga, NJ: Spectro-Chrome Inst., 1933).

11. D. Dinshah, *Let There Be Light* (Malaga, NJ: Dinshah Health Society, 1985).

12. E.O. Sterzer, from *Bulletin of the College of Syntonic Optometry* (Jan. 1936).

13. H.R. Spitler, *The Syntonic Principle* (College of Syntonic Optometry, 1941).

14. E.O. Sterzer, from *Bulletin of College of Syntonic Optometry* (Jan. 1936).

CHAPTER 7

1. Z. Kime, *Sunlight* (Penryn, CA: World Health Publications, 1980).

2. T.A. Brombach, *Visual Fields* (Transcript of lectures, 1936).

3. T.H. Eames, "Restrictions of the Visual Field as Handicaps to Learning," *Journal of Educational Research* 19 (Feb. 1936): pp. 460-463.

4. T.H. Eames, "The Speed of Picture Recognition and the Speed of Word Recognition in Cases of Reading Difficulty," *American Journal of Ophthalmology* 21 (Dec. 1938): pp. 1370-1375.

5. T.H. Eames, "The Relationship of the Central Visual Field to the Speed of Visual Perception," *American Journal of Ophthalmology* 43 (1957): pp. 279-280.

6. V.I. Shipman, "A Constriction of the Perceptual Field Under Stress" (Paper presented to the Eastern Psychol. Assoc., Philadelphia, PA, 1954).

7. M.D. Anderson and J.M. Williams, "Seeing Too Straight; Stress and Vision," *Longevity*, Aug. 1989.

8. "Noise Causes Bad Eyes," *Popular Science*, Apr. 1931, p. 33.

9. R. Kaplan, "Changes in Form Visual Fields in Reading Disabled Children Produced by Syntonic Stimulation," *International Journal of Biosocial Research* 5, no. 1 (1983): pp. 20-33.

10. J. Liberman, "The Effect of Syntonic Colored Light. Stimulation on Certain Visual and Cognitive Functions," *Journal of Optometric Vision Development* 17 (June 1986).

CHAPTER 8

1. H. Wohlfarth and Sam C. Wohlfarth, "The Effect of Color Psychodynamic Environmental Modification Upon Psychophysiological and Behavioral Reactions of Severely Handicapped Children," *The International Journal of Biosocial Research* 3, no. 1 (1982): pp. 10-38.

2. H. Ertel, *Kinder Farbstudien* 78 (München: Gesellschaft fur Rationale Psycholgie).

3. H. Wohlfarth and A. Schultz, "The Effect of Color Psychodynamic Environment Modification on Sound Noise Levels in Elementary Schools," *The International Journal of Biosocial Research* 5, no. 1 (1983): pp. 12-19.

4. H. Wohlfarth, "The Effects of Color-Psychodynamic Environmental Modification on Disciplinary Incidences in Elementary Schools Over One School Year: A Controlled Study," *The International Journal of Biosocial Research* 6, no. 1 (1984): pp. 44-53.

5. H. Wohlfarth, "The Effects of Color-Psychodynamic Environmental Modification on Absences Due to Illness in Elementary Schools: A Controlled Study," *The International Journal of Biosocial Research* 6, no. 1 (1984): pp. 54-61.

6. H. Wohlfarth, "The Effects of Color-Psychodynamic Environmental Color & Lighting Modification of Elementary Schools on Blood Pressure and Mood: A Controlled Study," *The International Journal of Biosocial Research* 7, no. 1 (1985): pp. 9-16.

7. H. Irlen, *Successful Treatment of Learning Disabilities* (Paper presented at the 91st Annual Convention of the American Psychological Assoc., Anaheim, CA, Aug. 1983).

8. P. Whiting, "How Difficult Can Reading Be? New Insights Into Reading Problems," *Journal of English Teacher's Association* 49 (Oct. 1985): pp. 49-55.

9. P. Whiting, "Improvements in Reading and Other Skills Using Irlen Colored Lenses," *Australian Journal of Remedial Education* 20 (1987): pp. 13-15.

10. G.L. Robinson, *Improvements in Reading Skills Using Irlen Colored Lenses: A Replication Survey* (Unpublished manuscript, Newcastle: Hunter Inst. of Higher Education).

11. G. Hannell et al., "Reading Improvement with Tinted Lenses: A Report of Two Cases," *Clinical and Experimental Optometry* 72.5 (Sept./Oct. 1989).

CHAPTER 9

1. J.N. Ott, "Color and Light: Their Effects on Plants, Animals, and People," *Journal of Biosocial Research* 7, part I (1985).

2. Ibid.

3. J. Sonneborn-Smith, "DNA Repair and Longevity Assurance in Paramecium Tetraurelia," *Science* 203, Mar. 16, 1979, pp. 1115-1117.

4. J. Sonneborn-Smith, "Aging in Protozoa," *Review of Biological Research in Aging* 1 (1983): pp. 29-35.

5. J. Sonneborn-Smith, "Genetics and Aging in Protozoa," *International Review of Cytology* 73 (1983).

6. C. Raab, "Uber die Wirkung Fluoreszirenden Stoffe auf Infusoria," *Z Biol.* 39 (1900): p. 534.

7. T.J. Dougherty, "The Bright Lights of Laser," *The Saturday Evening Post*, Dec. 1981, pp. 16-18, 120.

8. M. Shodell, "The Curative Light," *Science*, Apr. 1982, pp. 47-51.

9. Z. Kime, *Sunlight* (Penryn, CA: World Health Publications, 1980).

10. R.L. Lipson, E.J. Baldes, and A.M. Olson, "The Use of a Derivative of Hematoporphyrin in Tumor Detection," *Journal of National Cancer Institute* 26 (1961): pp. 1-8.

11. T.J. Dougherty et al., "Photoradiation Therapy II: Cure of Animal Tumors with Hematoporphyrin and Light," *Journal of National Cancer Institute* 55 (1975): p. 115.

12. T.J. Dougherty et al., "Photoradiation Therapy for the Treatment of Malignant Tumors," *Cancer Research* 38 (Aug. 1978): pp. 2628-2635.

13. T.J. Dougherty, "Hematoporphyrin Derivative for Detection and Treatment of Cancer," *Journal of Surgical Oncology* 15 (1980): pp. 209-210.

14. M. Moneysmith, "Lasers: New Light on Cancer," *The Saturday Evening Post*, Nov. 1981, pp. 52-55.

15. T.J. Dougherty, "Photoradiation Therapy—New Approaches," *Seminars in Surgical Oncology* 5 (1989): pp. 6-16.

16. M. Moneysmith, "Lasers: New Light on Cancer," *The Saturday Evening Post*, Nov. 1981, pp. 52-55.

17. E. Rosenthal, "Light-Sensitive Chemicals Join Arsenal of Anti-Cancer Weapons," *The New York Times*, Sept. 26, 1989, Medical Science section.

18. T.J. Dougherty, "Photosensitization of Malignant Tumors" (Reprint of book chapter to appear in *Adjuncts to Cancer Therapy*, ed. Steven Economou (Philadelphia: Lea & Febiger, 1990).

19. E. Rosenthal, op. cit.

20. M. Shodell, "The Curative Light," *Science*, Apr. 1982, pp. 47-51.

21. T.J. Dougherty, "Photoradiation Therapy—New Approaches," *Seminars in Surgical Oncology* 5 (1989): pp. 6-16.

22. Personal conversations with Dr. Thomas Dougherty in Jan. 1990.

23. E. Rosenthal, "Light-Sensitive Chemicals Join Arsenal of Anti-Cancer Weapons," *The New York Times*, Sept. 26, 1989, Medical Science section.

24. Personal conversations with Dr. Stuart Marcus, Deputy Director, Clinical Research, Oncology, in the Medical Research Division of American Cyanamid Company's Lederle Laboratories in Feb. 1990.

25. Personal conversations with Dr. Thomas Dougherty in Jan. 1990.

26. J. Graverholz, "SDI Lasers Inactivate the AIDS Virus: An Interview with Lester Mathews, Ph.D.," *Science and Technology* EIR (Jan. 29, 1988).

27. J.T. Newman et al., "Photodynamic Inactivation of Viruses and Its Application for Blood Banking," *Baylor University Medical Center Proceedings* 1, no. 2 (Apr. 1988): pp. 2-14.

28. M.M. Judy, "Photodynamic Inactivation of Viruses and Its Potential Application for Blood Banking," *Bio-Laser News* (Oct. 1989).

29. R. Engelman, "Light Kills AIDS Virus in Blood," *Scripps Howard News Service*, Jan. 13, 1988.

30. J. Graverholz, "SDI Lasers Inactivate the AIDS Virus: An Interview with Lester Mathews, Ph.D.," *Science and Technology* EIR (Jan. 29, 1988).

31. A. Ramirez, "A Star Wars Laser Comes to Earth," *Fortune*, Aug. 15, 1988.

CHAPTER 10

1. N.E. Rosenthal, *Seasons of the Mind* (New York: Bantam, 1989).

2. S. Rovner, "Treating SADness With Light," *Washington Post*, Sept. 19, 1989, Health section.

3. N.E. Rosenthal, and T.A. Wehr, "Seasonal Affective Disorders," *Psychiatric Annals* 17, no. 10 (Oct. 1987): pp. 670-674.

4. N.E. Rosenthal, *Seasons of the Mind* (New York: Bantam, 1989).

5. J.F. Cauvin, *Des Bienfaits de L'Insolation* (Paris: 1815).

6. A. Lewy et al., "Light Suppresses Melatonin Secretion in Humans," *Science* 210, 1980, pp. 1267-1269.

7. N.E. Rosenthal et al., "Seasonal Affective Disorder: A Description of the Syndrome and Preliminary Findings With Light Therapy," *Archives General Psychiatry* 41 (1984): pp. 72-80.

8. M. Cross, "New Techniques Help Cure Winter Blues," *The Valley Vantage*, Feb. 1, 1990, p. 5.

9. N.E. Rosenthal, *Brain/Mind Bulletin* 11, no. 13 (July 1986): p. 3.

10. M. Terman et al., *Brain/Mind Bulletin* 15, no. 5, (Feb. 1990): p. 3.

11. M. Terman et al., "Dawn and Dusk Simulation as a Therapeutic Intervention," *Biological Psychiatry* 25 (1989): pp. 966-970.

12. N.E. Rosenthal, *Seasons of the Mind* (New York: Bantam, 1989).

13. P. Mueller and R. Davies, *Brain/Mind Bulletin* 11, no. 11 (June 16, 1986): p. 2.

14. D.F. Kripke, "Therapeutic Effects of Bright Light in Depression," *Annals of New York Academy of Science* 453 (1985): pp. 270-281.

15. N.E. Rosenthal, *Seasons of the Mind* (New York: Bantam, 1989).

16. "Alcohol Treatment Helped by Light Treatment," *Nutrition Health Review*, Fall 1988.

17. I. Geller, *International Journal of Biosocial Research* 8, Special Subject Issue (1986): pp. 65-66.

18. R.J. Reiter, "Light as a Drug" (Lecture presented at the 56th Annual College of Syntonic Optometry Conference, Estes Park, CO, May 1988).

19. R.J. Reiter, "The Pineal Gland: An Important Link to the Environment," *NIPS* 1 (Dec. 1986): pp. 202-205.

20. I. Geller, *International Journal of Biosocial Research* 8, Special Subject Issue (1986): pp. 65-66.

21. Ibid.

22. Ibid.

23. C.A. Czeisler et al., "Bright Light Induction of Strong (Type O) Resetting of Human Circadian Pacemaker," *Science* 244, pp. 1328-1332.

24. R. Pool, "Illuminating Jet Lag," *Science* 244, pp. 1256-1257.

25. S. Campbell et al., *Brain/Mind Bulletin* 14, no. 4 (Jan. 1989): p. 8.

26. M. Jenkins, "Jet Lag Breakthrough: The Key is When to Turn on the Bright Light," *The Condé Nast Traveler*, Sept. 1989, pp. 35-36.

27. J. Gross and L. Malcmacher, "Advances in Denture Reline," *Dentistry Today*.

28. Personal conversations with Dr. Joshua Friedman, Demetron Research Corp., in Jan. 1990.

29. R. Gerber, *Vibrational Medicine* (Santa Fe, NM: Bear & Co., 1988).

30. Personal conversations and correspondence with Dr. Hazel Parcells in Jan. 1990.

31. R.E. Frenkel, "Controlling Human Stress by Imageoscopy," *The Journal for Better Living*, Summer 1985.

32. R.E. Frenkel, "Light Therapy: The Prevention, Control, and Treatment of Suicide," *The Journal for Better Living*, Spring 1987.

33. Personal conversations and correspondence with Dr. Richard Frenkel as adapted from his forthcoming book, tentatively entitled *Overcoming Stress*.

34. B.L. Parry et al., "Morning Versus Evening Bright Light Treatment of Late Luteal Phase Dysphoric Disorder," *American Journal of Psychiatry* 146 (Sept. 1989): p. 9.

35. Rainbow Canyon, personal correspondence with author, Feb. 1990.

36. Tolbert McCarroll, *Notes From the Song of Life* (Berkeley: Celestial Arts, 1977, 1987), p. 17.

CHAPTER 11

1. E. Caldwell, "Liquid Sunglasses," *Hippocrates*, Nov./Dec. 1989.

2. A.P. Zabaluyeva, "The Mechanism of Adaptiogenic Effect of Ultraviolet," *Vestn. Akad. Med. Nauk.* 3 (1975): p. 23.

3. G. Frick, "Effect of UV of Blood on Blood Picture," *Folia Haemat* 101 (1974): p. 871.

4. F. Hollwich, *The Influence of Ocular Light Perception on Metabolism in Man and in Animal* (New York: Springer-Verlag, 1979).

5. J.N. Ott, "Color and Light: Their Effects on Plants, Animals, and People," *Journal of Biosocial Research* 7, part I (1985).

6. Z. Kime, *Sunlight* (Penryn, CA: World Health Publications, 1980).

7. *The Swannanoa Health Report*, issues 2 & 3 (Charlottesville, VA: Swannanoa Institute, Ltd., 1989): p. 2.

8. A. Armagnal, "Finds Ways to Tune Rays of Ultra Violet," *Popular Science Monthly*, Apr. 1931, pp. 42-43, 132-133.

9. M.F. Holick and M.B. Clark, "The Photobiogenesis and Metabolism and Vitamin D," *Fed. Proc.* 37 (1978): p. 2567.

10. M.F. Holick et al., "Advances in the Photobiology of Vitamin D-3," (Second Annual Scientific Meeting of the American Society for Bone and Mineral Research, Washington, D.C., U.S.A., June 16-17, 1980) *CALCIF Tissue International* 31, no. 1, p. 79.

11. M.F. Holick et al., "Photosynthesis of Previtamin D-3 in Human Skin and the Physiologic Consequences," *Science* 210, Oct. 10, 1980, pp. 203-205.

12. M.F. Holick, J.A. MacLaughlin, and S.H. Doppelt, "Regulation of Cutaneous Previtamin D-3 Photosynthesis in Man: Skin Pigment Is Not An Essential Regulator," *Science* 211, Feb. 6, 1981, pp. 590-593.

13. J.A. MacLaughlin, R.R. Anderson, and M.F. Holick, "Spectral Character of Sunlight Modulates Photosynthesis of Previtamin D-3 and Its Photoisomers in Human Skin," *Science* 216, May 28, 1982, pp. 1001-1003.

14. R.M. Neer et al., "Stimulation by Artificial Lighting of Calcium Absorption in Elderly Human Subjects," *Nature* 229 (1971): p. 255.

15. J.R. Johnson, "The Effect of Carbon Arc Radiation on Blood Pressure and Cardiac Output," *American Journal of Physiology* 114 (1935): p. 594.

16. Ibid.

17. L. Lohmeier, "Let the Sun Shine In," *East West*, July 1986, pp. 36-39.

18. L.A. Kunitsina et al., "Therapeutic Action of Ultraviolet Irradiation in a Complex Treatment of Patients with Initial Cerebral Atherosclerosis," *Sovet Med* 33 (1970): p. 89.

19. V.A. Mikhailov, "Influence of Graduated Sunlight Baths on Patients with Coronary Atherosclerosis," *Sovet Med* 29 (1966): p. 76.

20. A.I. Pertsovskij et al., "Preventive Activity of Ultraviolet Rays in the Presence of Experimental Atherosclerosis," *Vop Kurort Fizioter* 36 (1971): p. 203.

21. R. Altschul and I.H. Herman, "Ultraviolet Irradiation and Cholesterol Metabolism; Seventh Annual Meeting of The American Society for the Study of Arteriosclerosis," *Circulation* 8 (1953): p. 438.

22. L. Lohmeier, "Let the Sun Shine In," *East West*, July 1986, pp. 36-39.

23. Ibid.

24. I.I. Belyayev et al., "Combined Use of Ultraviolet Radiation to Control Acute Respiratory Disease," *Vestn Akad Med Nauk SSSR* 3 (1975): p. 37.

25. N.M. Dantsig, "Ultraviolet Radiation," in Russian language book (Moscow: 1966).

26. A.P. Zabaluyeva, "General Immunological Reactivity of the Organism in Prophylactic Ultraviolet Irradiation of Children in Northern Regions," *Vestn Akad Med Nauk* 3 (1975): p. 23.

27. T.K. Das Gupta and J. Terz, "Influence of Pineal Gland on the Growth and Spread of Melanoma in the Hamster," *Cancer Research* 27 (1967): p. 1306.

28. W. Stumpf et al., *Brain/Mind Bulletin* 15, no. 1 (Oct. 1989): p. 2.

29. This and other portions of this chapter were adapted from *The Swannanoa Health Report*, issues 2 and 3, entitled, "The Miraculous Health Benefits of Ultraviolet Light!" For information on Health Discoveries Newsletter, please write to: 612 Rio Road West, Charlottesville, VA 22901.

30. J.N. Ott, "Color and Light: Their Effects on Plants, Animals, and People," *Journal of Biosocial Research* 7, part I (1985).

31. Ibid.

32. W.T. Ham et al., "Action Spectrum for Retinal Injury From Near-Ultraviolet Radiation in the Aphakic Monkey," *American Journal of Ophthalmology* (Mar. 1982).

33. J.N. Ott, "Color and Light: Their Effects on Plants, Animals, and People," *Journal of Biosocial Research* 7, part I (1985).

34. Z. Kime, *Sunlight* (Penryn, CA: World Health Publications, 1980).

35. John Marshall, "Light and the Ageing Eye," *The RSA Journal* 138, no. 5406 (May 1990): 406-418.

36. V. Beral et al., "Malignant Melanoma and Exposure to Fluorescent Light at Work," *Lancet* 2 (1982): pp. 290-292.

37. B.S. Pasternak, N. Dubin, & M. Moseson, "Malignant Melanoma and Exposure to Fluorescent Light at Work," *Lancet* 1 (1983): p. 704.

38. D.S. Rigel et al., "Malignant Melanoma and Exposure to Fluorescent Lighting at Work," *Lancet* 1 (1983): p. 704.

39. W. Allen, "Suspected Carcinogen Found in 14 of 17 Sunscreens," *St. Louis Post Dispatch*, Mar. 9, 1989.

CHAPTER 12

1. J.N. Ott, *Light Radiation and You* (Greenwich, CT: Devin-Adair Publishers, 1982).

2. J.N. Ott, "Color and Light: Their Effects on Plants, Animals, and People, Part 4," *International Journal of Biosocial Research* 10, Special Subject Issue (1988): pp. 111-116, 126, 127.

CHAPTER 13

1. F. Popp, *Brain/Mind Bulletin* 10, no. 14 (Aug. 19, 1985): p. 1.

2. H. Pohl, *Brain/Mind Bulletin* 10, no. 14 (Aug. 19, 1985): p. 1.

3. P. Narendra, *Brain/Mind Bulletin* 9, no. 9 (May 7, 1984): p. 2.

4. D. Cooper, "The Physics of Light," *College of Syntonic Optometry Journal* (Mar. 1990): p. 2.

5. D. Ullman, *Homeopathy: Medicine for the 21st Century* (Berkeley, CA: North Atlantic Books, 1988).

6. R. Leviton, "Homeopathy," *Yoga Journal*, issue 85, Mar./Apr. 1989, pp. 42-51, 97-99, 105.

7. Ibid.

CHAPTER 14

1. T. Bearden, "AIDS: Urgent Comments on Mankind's Greatest Threat and the Secrets of Electromagnetic Healing," *Journal of the U.S. Psychotronics Association* 1, no. 1 (Nov. 1988).

2. Bartholomew, *I Come As A Brother* (Taos, NM: High Mesa Press, 1984), pp. 38-39.

SUGGESTED READING

Amber, R.B. *Color Therapy*. New York: Samuel Weiser, Inc., 1964.

Babbitt, Edwin S. *The Principles of Light and Color*. Secaucus, NJ: Citadel Press, 1967.

Bandler, Richard and John Grinder. *Frogs Into Princes*. Moab, UT: Real People Press, 1979.

Birren, Faber. *Color Psychology & Color Healing*. Secaucus, NJ: Citadel Press, 1961.

Brain/Mind Bulletin. Los Angeles: Interface Press.

Brennan, Barbara Ann. *Hands of Light*. New York: Bantam, 1987.

Cousens, Gabriel. *Spiritual Nutrition and the Rainbow Diet*. Boulder, CO: Cassandra Press, 1986.

Dinshah, Darius. *Let There Be Light*. Malaga, NJ: Dinshah Health Society, 1985.

Frieling, Heinrich. *The Color Mirror*. Zurich-Frankfurt: Musterschmidt Göttingen, 1975.

Gerber, Richard. *Vibrational Medicine*. Santa Fe, NM: Bear and Co., 1988.

Ghadiali, Dinshah, P. *Spectro-Chrome Metry Encyclopedia*. Malaga, NJ: Spectro-Chrome Institute, 1933.

Gimbel, Theo. *Healing Through Color*. Great Britain: The C.W. Daniel Company, Ltd., 1980.

Greenberg, Michael A. *Off the Pedestal: Transforming the Business of Medicine*. Houston: Breakthru Publishing, 1990.

Hills, Christopher. *Nuclear Evolution*. Boulder Creek, CA: University of the Trees Press, 1977.

Hills, Norah. *You Are a Rainbow*. Boulder Creek, CA: University of the Trees Press, 1979.

Hollwich, Fritz. *The Influence of Ocular Light Perception on Metabolism in Man and in Animal*. New York: Springer-Verlag, 1979.

Hunt, Roland. *The Seven Keys to Color Healing*. San Francisco: Harper & Row, 1971.

Kaplan, Robert-Michael. *Seeing Beyond 20/20*. Hillsboro, OR: Beyond Words Publishing, 1987.

Lüscher, Max. *The Lüscher Color Test*. New York: Washington Square Press, 1969.

McWilliams, Charles H. *Electro Acupuncture Up To Date*. USA: Health Sciences Research, 1981.

Ott, John N. *Health and Light*. Old Greenwich, CT: The Devin-Adair Co., 1973.

Ott, John N. *Light Radiation and You*. Greenwich, CT: The Devin-Adair Co., 1982.

Ott, John N. *My Ivory Cellar*. Chicago: Twentieth Century Press, Inc., 1958.

Ouseley, S.G.J. *The Power of the Rays*. London: L.N. Fowler & Co., Ltd., 1951.

Reiter, R.J. and M. Karasek. *Advances in Pineal Research*. Vol. 1. London-Paris: John Libbey, 1986.

Robbins, John. *Diet for a New America*. Walpole, NH: Stillpoint Publishing, 1987.

Rosenthal, Norman E. *Seasons of the Mind*. New York: Bantam, 1989.

Russell, Walter. *The Secret of Light*. Waynesboro, VA: University of Science and Philosophy, Swannanoa, 1974.

Schwarz, Jack. *Human Energy Systems*. New York: E.P. Dutton, 1980.

Steiner, Rudolf. *Colour*. London: Rudolf Steiner Press, 1982.

Swannanoa Health Report. Swannanoa Institute, Ltd. 612 Rio Road West, Charlottesville, VA 22901.

Trexler, Gary. *The World of Light, Color, Health, and Behavior*. Fairfield, IA: self-published, 1985.

Wood, Betty. *The Healing Power of Color*. New York: Destiny Books, 1984.

Wurtman, Richard J., Michael J. Baum and John T. Potts, Jr. *The Medical and Biological Effects of Light*. New York: The New York Academy of Sciences, 1985.

Exploring the Spectrum. Parts I & II. A film by John Ott.

INDEX

243

X, Y, Z

ABOUT THE AUTHOR

Dr. Jacob Liberman is considered a pioneer in the therapeutic use of light and color and the art of mind/body integration. He attended the University of Georgia, earned a doctorate in optometry (O.D.) in 1973, and received a Ph.D. in vision science in 1986 for his pioneering work in phototherapy. Since 1973 he has lectured extensively throughout the United States and Europe and has been published in both professional and popular journals.

Integrating scientific research, clinical experience, and his own intuitive insights, Dr. Liberman has worked effectively with more than 30,000 individuals, ranging from the learning disabled and physically/emotionally traumatized to business executives and Olympic athletes.

Dr. Liberman is immediate past president of the College of Syntonic Optometry, an organization of optometrists and other health professionals that has advocated the use of light therapy by way of the eyes since its founding in the 1930s. He is also president of Universal Light Technologies, Ltd., a company researching and developing phototherapeutic devices for healing.

For information regarding lectures, workshops,
and products for personal healing, contact:

Jacob Liberman, O.D., Ph.D.
Universal Light Technology
P.O. Box 520
Carbondale, CO 81623
Toll-Free Ordering: 800-81-LIGHT
Phone 303-927-0100   Fax 303-927-0101

BOOKS OF RELATED INTEREST
BY BEAR & COMPANY

ACCEPTING YOUR POWER TO HEAL
The Personal Practice of Therapeutic Touch
by Dolores Krieger, Ph.D., R.N.

BREATHING
Expanding Your Power and Energy
by Michael Sky

ECSTASY IS A NEW FREQUENCY
Teachings of The Light Institute
by Chris Griscom

EMERGENCE OF THE DIVINE CHILD
Healing the Emotional Body
by Rick Phillips

LIQUID LIGHT OF SEX
Understanding Your Key Life Passages
by Barbara Hand Clow

VIBRATIONAL MEDICINE
New Choices for Healing Ourselves
by Richard Gerber, M.D.

WHY DON'T I FEEL BETTER?
Healing the Recovering Alcoholic
by Joyce Bismack

Contact your local bookseller or write:
BEAR & COMPANY
P.O. Drawer 2860
Santa Fe, NM 87504